Chemo Induced Insanity

Carol A. Goad

INFINITY PUBLISHING

ISBN 978-0-7414-6953-3

Printed in the United States of America

Published October 2012

INFINITY PUBLISHING

Toll-free (877) BUY BOOK
Local Phone (610) 941-9999
Fax (610) 941-9959
Info@buybooksontheweb.com
www.buybooksontheweb.com

Dedicated to

Our God
My rock, My shelter in the storm, My Savior

To my husband Travis,
Thank you for loving me, putting up with me, and for encouraging me.

To my five angels sent from God himself
Nychelle, Brice, Alexandria, Alaina, and Noah
Thank you for being strong and pulling together when mom and dad need you.

And last but not least to our parents for always being there especially when it's critical,
our family and friends who pray for us,
our home church Destiny for holding us close and loving us like family,
and to our little community of BIG DIAMOND for showing heart and love to your neighbors.
Thank you all!

"Today you are going into battle
against your enemies.
Do not be faint hearted or afraid;
Do not be terrified or give way to
panic before them.
For the Lord your God
is the one who goes with you
to fight for you against your enemies
to give you victory."

Deuteronomy 20:3-4

This was my battle cry.

One day things are going along ok.
The next day something changes.

The Pink Ribbons.

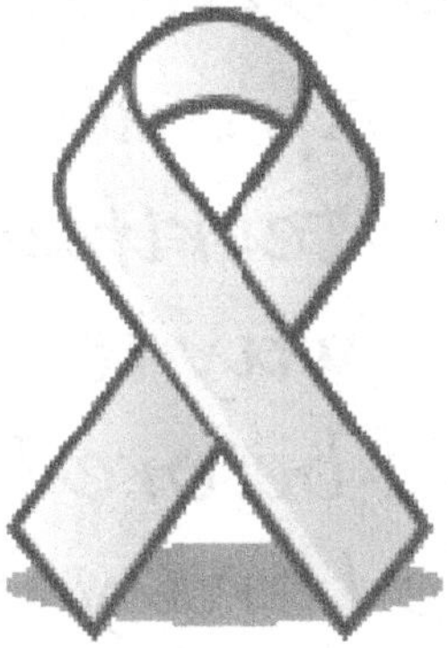

They are everywhere.
Until you are personally touched by breast cancer by either being diagnosed yourself
or knowing someone close to you
who has been diagnosed, you don't *really* see them.

I didn't really notice them before.

Now I can't *help* but notice them.

Everybody has their story don't they? I'm inclined to leave some of mine out. This is mostly because we have heard it all before. You know how it goes, "I felt a lump, went to the doctor – cancer – blah blah blah – chemo – blah – removal of breast – Whoa! Stop right there! We don't just go slicing and dicing of the girls just because someone said the big bad scary word

………….. CANCER!

Okay, maybe I will go ahead and tell my story.

I can at least tell the important and fun parts.

Prologue

Cancer has become so prevalent that almost everyone knows someone who had it, has it, or has lost their battle to it.

It shows up on your doorstep usually with no warning. My first experience with cancer was when my grandmother had it. She had ovarian cancer that spread through her body like wildfire.

My memory is fuzzy about that moment in my life. It was the 80's and I was in my early teens. What my mind remembers is that grandma fought hard and then it seems in the snap of a finger, she was gone. I want you to know my grandmother was an amazing person. She was a fighter. She had 10 children and raised them all into adulthood. She went through some incredible circumstances and pushed through. She was a true warrior, and we miss her very much.

Cancer is UGLY.

That's how cancer is sometimes.
It rears its ugly head and you fight and pray.
Sometimes you win.

In the year leading up to my diagnosis, the year of my treatment, and the year and a half after hearing I was cancer free (this is about the time I begin writing this book); I watched a friend fight cancer and win, a close family friend die of lung cancer, two uncles diagnosed within a couple months of each other fight and win their battle with prostate cancer, and my father-in-law lose his battle with bladder cancer.

These are people I know personally. Not friends of friends.

My point in telling you all of this is to ask you to just be aware of the people around you and their personal fight with it. Be aware of what you're eating, and how it affects your body. Be aware of the government regulations regarding our food. And be aware of your own bodies. Know what is normal and what isn't.

You hear it time and time again, but a lot of the time it doesn't really sink in.

~ EARLY DETECTION
IS IMPERATIVE FOR
SURVIVAL
WHEN DEALING WITH CANCER.

Some of the excerpts in this book are from an actual blog my mother-in-law set up for me when I was sick. Whenever the urge struck me, I would write in it as I fought my own battle with breast cancer.

You may be reading this because you have just been diagnosed (Hey, don't look back, put your seat belt on, pedal to the metal, you CAN beat this!), or you may be in the middle of it (everyday that you wake up, opening your eyes and realizing your still here is a gift. Keep Fighting!), or you may be on the other side, with cancer in your rear view mirror (paranoia NOT allowed! I mean with as many drugs that have been through your system, nothing survived!) The good news is that no matter what your reason, *hope abounds!* Rest your spirit. Let yourself smile, and *remember to laugh!* It really is the best medicine!

"Thank you GOD
for carrying me when I couldn't walk and
for being my strength when all I felt was weakness."

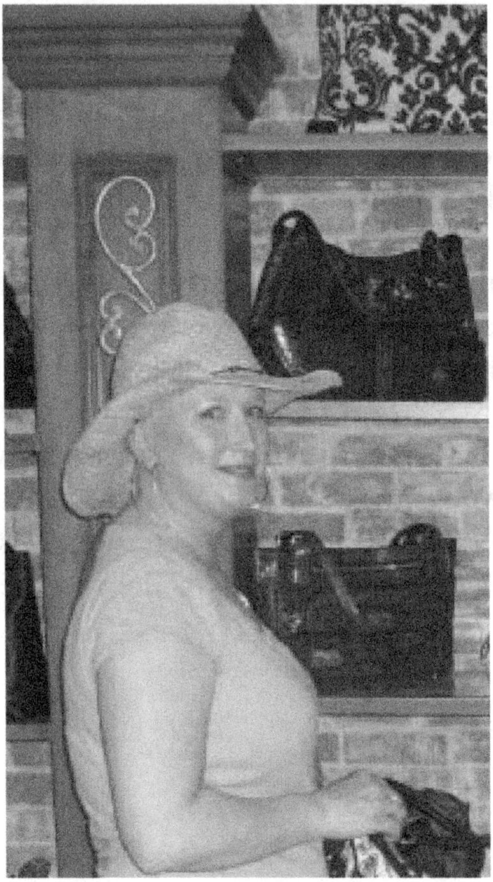

Me in 2008
In the middle of my treatment.

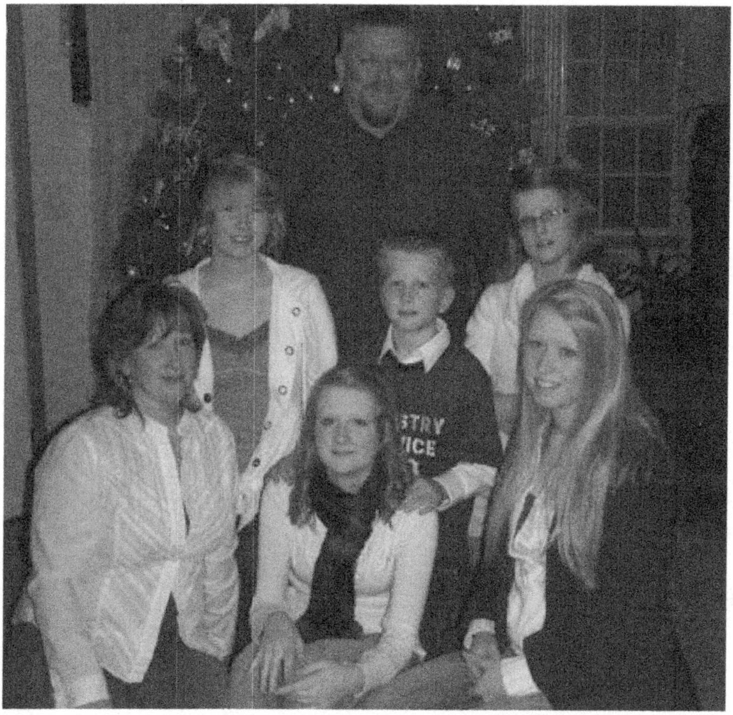

Our Family Christmas 2009

My Story

(My version)

You know, because I was only 35, the thought of doing a self exam didn't really cross my mind. And even if I did do one, I really had no idea of what I was looking for anyway! Hindsight is 20/20 though, as they say. If you feel something that's not supposed to be there, you just know it's not right.

In October of '07, I was lying in bed when I felt this itchy stinging sensation on the left side of my left breast, almost under my arm. When I scratched though, the scratching was met with an almost prickling sensation. My first thought was "That was weird." And then "What the heck could have bit me in October?" Now at this point, I decide I have to "see" this source of irritation. Upon closer inspection I did not find anything I could "see". I ran my fingers over the itchy spot again and pressed in a little. This time, I felt a little round bump. It sort of reminded me of a small marble. I wasn't sure what to think about it.

I decided it wasn't much to worry about. For one, I was only 35! I'm young! And two, I'm always hearing about calcium deposits and fibroids that are harmless and nothing to fret over. So I'm sure that if it's anything at all, it's one of those.

The next few weeks there was some pain and it would come and go. I really just let it slip to the back of my mind. This was a busy month that led into more busy months. We were two weeks from Halloween and I had costumes to get done! I do remember that there were a couple of times that it was almost painful to put on or take off my shirt. I still had no idea what to think about all of that. I had other things going on and no time to deal with this. Looking back I can see that I just became really preoccupied. On November 2nd my 57 year old dad passed away unexpectedly of a massive heart attack. If you can picture Popeye, you will see my dad, muscles and all, only better looking. He was healthy. It was a shock. Something that was not possible. God had different plans I guess.

The next four months became a bit of a blur. Through all of that, I didn't give that lump much of a thought.

Sometime around the first part of January, things started to slow a little bit. I was standing in the shower one morning and remembered "it". So, really just out of curiosity, I checked to see if it was still there. It was. Only now, it was different.

Over the next few weeks I kind of kept my eye on it. I was vaguely aware of some pain. It came and went. It did seem to be growing. Or was it my imagination? Somewhere towards the end of January I decide to have my husband weigh in on this "thing".

I'm not crazy! He agrees that there is something there. A couple of weeks later I ask him if he thinks it's growing. His response is "BABE! You have to go get that checked out!" I roll my eyes, and with just a drop of sarcasm I say "OK! I'll get right on that." You see I'm not a "run to the doctor every time I'm sick" kind of person. I think the last time I actually went to see a doctor was eight years prior when I gave birth to my son.

Around the first part of February, my family and I were all standing in the kitchen conversing about this and that. (This is where all important conversations happen in our house. We have nearly solved the Health Care crisis in that very room!) During the course of a conversation that was about a mom in our community and her fight with cancer, for some reason, I decide to say something about this lump. It was out of my mouth before I could stop it. My step-mom and oldest (16 yr old) daughter got a little upset. They wanted me to call the very next day to make an appointment. I assured them so I thought, that I had done a little research and that there was nothing to worry about. A week or so prior, I looked up calcium deposits and felt there was nothing I should worry about.

There are very few secrets in our house. There are kids, family, and friends coming and going constantly. So it is a little hard to keep things quiet. My sixteen year old daughter, she is my worrier, after a week of reminding me to call the doctor and make an appointment, decides she needs to enlist my 14 year old daughter and bring her in for back up.

You see my 14 year old can be a bit of a drill sergeant. She likes things done a certain way and orderly. A lot of times she doesn't mind letting you know if things aren't in order. I have no doubt that if she joined the military she would be sitting in the White House just inside a few years of duty. Brice (my 14 yr old) marches right up to me like a mother ready to scold a child. My 16 year old is right behind her. Brice almost barks at me "MOM! Do you have a lump?" I stand there stunned by her tone of voice toward me, the fact that she is still moving toward me, and feeling like I am in deep trouble, I stammer "Wh-What?" I ask. Actually, I heard her. I was trying to come up with a quick witty response. She repeats herself with a look that says "You're going down!"

I laugh. It's my first line of defense. Ask my kids. When I am trying to discipline them, they know if they find a way to make me laugh it's all over with. On the other hand, in this sort of situation I think it really annoys my family. With a little playful attitude I say "Yeah! So? You gotta problem with it call my lawyer!" This kind of retort almost always works. They hate that. Brice softens a little and says "Seriously, mom, you have to go see a doctor." I look over her shoulder, making eye contact with Nychelle (my 16 year old), and ask Brice "Who told you anyway?" Nychelle confirms what I already know. She says "I told her mom, you said you were going to go to the doctor last week!" Brice then calls in re-enforcements. "Dad! Do you know mom has a lump?"

By this time my step-mom has heard the commotion and has come into the room. I feel like I'm about to be in the middle of a scary confrontation. As my husband comes into the room I smile, glad he has known and that he is going to be on my side. "Yes." he says "I have been telling her to go see the doctor."

So much for having an ally.

The rest of the conversation is inconsequential. I stood there smiling and rolling my eyes. I give in, throw my hands into the air and say "Fine! If you people will quit crying and whining about it, I will call and make an appointment so that I can be poked and prodded so that you will all feel better. Ok?"

I knew they had formed a sort of alliance against me, so I knew I had to follow through. I have to tell you, how proud I am of my family, having gone through that scene in my mind many times. We have our son and four girls . God bless that little boys' heart. He has grown up hearing arguments about who is wearing what shirt or who borrowed what pair of jeans without asking. But when it's important, they pull together and form a team that would be hard to beat.

I call to make an appointment. Guess what? They can get me in quick! Oh joy. I can't wait. (Again sarcasm) About three days later I am at my regular doctor for an exam. They tell me they do feel something and to be double sure it's nothing to worry about, they are going to set me up an appointment for a mammogram. It's standard when finding something like this. My appointment is for 3 days later at the Womens' Center. At this point I still feel invincible. I know it's all just routine.

I get to the Women's Center, and get signed in. This will be my first mammogram. All those e-mails about what happens during this kind of test are going through my mind. The only word that keeps reappearing is "smash". I just keep taking slow deep breaths. I am not really looking forward to letting the girls get "smashed". It sounds terrible and painful. Then I give myself a pep talk. "Listen Carol, you have had five kids. This is nothing. Quit being a big ol' baby." Did the pep talk work? Yes and no. Finally they take me back. It's funny, even though I have given birth to 5 children and have very little sense of modesty anymore; it is still very strange to have what feels like, anyone and their dog handling my breast. Were the e-mails right? Yes. It's sad but true. Do they spring back after being smashed? Well, I can't speak for everyone, but mine did. Thank goodness!

They tell me to have a seat and wait while the tech takes a quick look. I sit there wondering why they don't just let me go get dressed. It's freezing. The girl comes back and says "Do you have time to do an ultra sound?" She says "The tech thinks having an ultra sound will help rule a few things out". So I'm thinking, "Well, okay."

So during the ultra sound I am watching the monitor and the ultra sound techs face. Do you know that looking at a breast via ultra sound is kind of like looking at a deep sea ocean critter? Yep. It is. I made small talk with her. I tried to get her to tell me what she thought, but man they are hard to crack! When she finished she said "Give me just a second and let me bring the doctor in." So again, I am laying there half naked, freezing. I look to my left and wonder why there are two dressing rooms in a room that can only accommodate one person. I also realize I am really high off the ground. I make a mental note not to squirm too much. It would be embarrassing to explain why I was rushed to the hospital topless.

The Ultrasound (u.s.) Tech comes back in with the doctor. He explains they see something that is suspicious. (NO KIDDING?) Inside, I laugh. He tells me that they need to do a biopsy. They explain what it entails and asks if I have time to do that or they can set up another appointment. I'm thinking, "Well we are already here, let's make a day of it! Maybe later I can justify having a triple scoop in a sugar cone for having to go through *so much.*" The u.s. tech goes to find the biopsy tech. She assures me he is "really good". Awesome.

They come back and start prepping me for this biopsy. They used the ultra sound to help guide the biopsy needle. It was actually kind of cool to watch. It wasn't painful, just maybe odd. There was a clicking sound for each sample. When it was over they patted me on the head, told me I was a good girl and gave me a cool band-aid and a sticker. I'm just kidding. I did get a gauze pad with fun white tape and an appointment to come back to get the results the following week.

At this point I am starting to feel a little anxious, but I'm not necessarily feeling worried. During the four day wait for the results of the biopsy, I decided to do a little research on breast cancer and all the things it entails. I also tried to dig up a little more information about fibroids and calcium deposits. I learned a lot. I chose to believe that what I had was calcium deposits. I felt there was nothing to worry about. Calcium deposits are apparently a very common thing.

The day of my appointment came. I was either so sure of what they were going to tell me, or I was in complete denial.

My daughter and one of her friends were sitting in the waiting room. My husband came with me this time, "Just in case I need him" he said. We were brought back into a room. The doctor was very forth right with my results. I guess there are not really a lot of ways to tell someone they have cancer.

He said "Well, we have your results and the best way to go at it sometimes is to just get it out there." He said "They did find it to be malignant. This means it is not good. What it looks like is Invasive Ductal Carcinoma."

Well, okay. I sat there just slightly shaking my head up and down. I was trying to memorize all the important words. At that point I wasn't upset. I think it was more shock. I mean what he just said, doesn't sound anything like calcium deposits. I just looked at my husband, and give him a half hearted "well, how do you like them apples" kind of smile. He looked at me with concern. Actually he looks at me with concern on a regular basis. The doctor then proceeded to lightly skim over some options to "think about". These were things such as partial mastectomy or a full mastectomy. I thought, "Whoa, just a minute." I went from "Ok, this is not a big deal, I'll probably have to take a pill" to......waving sharp things around!

I feel a little dazed. He gives me a stack of papers and tells me to stop at the front desk and make an appointment to see him at his office in a week. I stopped at the front desk and did as I was told.

Have you ever had one of those moments that time kind of slows down in an instant, and then all of a sudden it catches back up? Yeah, that's what happened to me in that moment in time. One of the nurses came over and handed me a folder with all kinds of information in it. She then went through what was in there, such as surgery, chemo therapy, and radiation. She also went through the next steps I needed to take, and the things I needed to be thinking about before going to see the surgeon the following week.

I'm not ashamed to admit, I cried, right there at the appointment desk.

I think I cried most at the thought of removing a breast. I mean do you know how long girls wait for those things to show up? Some girls even stuff their bras until the day they can fill them on their own!

This is a big deal.

A Week To Make A Major Decision

Travis and I went home feeling a little lost. What I really wanted to do was to just ignore it and hope it disappears. Things disappear in our house all the time. All I needed to do was to push it to the side and wha-la! The Not-Me fairy will take care of it! I see it happen on a regular basis. My husband wouldn't hear of it. I can't express to you how he annoyed me. He has never been a sit back and let things happen kind of guy. He is a planner. I am not. So, all I hear is "Call your doctor, call your mom, call my friends wife, blah blah blah". All I could think was "You are SERIOUSLY disturbing my plan to sweep this under the rug!!"

I decide I'm going to read and soak up all the info I can about what I do know. This way I can make a better informed decision. We live in a very small community. The news I had cancer had reached everyone in less time than it took me to learn about it! A friend of ours who learned about my diagnosis through their children, called a few days later.

She gave me some fantastic advice. She said "Do not get into a hurry and make rash decisions." She told us that we needed to at least get a second opinion. She said "Find a cancer center in a larger city that specializes in just cancer. Go talk to them and hear what they have to say. Then make your decisions." That phone call calmed me to some degree. She made me feel like I was in control. I felt like I had a second to breath and think. We did as she advised. I don't think there is anything I could say or do that would show her how much I truly appreciate her. (THANK YOU LISA!) I feel as if she is one of my own personal angels. That little bit of advice changed the course of my treatment for the better.

March 12th we drove the over 2 hour drive to Kansas University Medical Center to meet with an oncologist there. We brought with us all my tests and paperwork from our local hospital and doctor. We were so pleased with everyone there and how we were treated. Everyone seemed as if they were there for me only. It seems as if there was no question they couldn't answer or at least find an answer to.

What I found out that day was that the kind of cancer I had was called Triple Negative Breast Cancer. What that means is that the three receptors that the cancer feeds off of is negative of certain hormones in my cancer. So I guess basically they don't know what exactly feeds this type of cancer. At least this is the way I understand it. Triple Negative Cancer is apparently a very aggressive cancer. As a result they did not want to delay in starting chemo.

We started for the over two hour ride back home. I think we were both feeling like we had been punched in the gut. I didn't sign up for this chemo junk. There is no telling what they put through your veins! I read somewhere that your body has only so many healing cards that you can cash in. It is then all downhill from there. I don't know if that's true or not, but I'm a little scared I am fixing to cash in my whole deck. I hope I don't get sick again after this!

March 17th would be our next trip to K.C. I will start chemo. NOW I'm a little scared.

Day

by

Day

The following pages will have my blog entries in *Italics*. I did correct some typos when preparing them for this book, but for the most part I left them as I wrote them. Sometimes I wrote them late at night or early in the morning. A lot of times I was under the influence of treatment drugs. So, please read accordingly.

My sweet mom-in-law started a blog for me to keep family and friends updated.

The following is her first entry;

Monday, March 17th 2008   03:48 pm

Carol is meeting this crisis head on and has a lot of courage. Her first treatment today was four hours long. Her legs have become weak. She is being brought back by her husband, but will be returning again tomorrow.

These are my mom-in-laws next few journal entries. She is so sweet! I was not yet in a place to start writing, so she was doing great in keeping everyone updated.

Tuesday, March 18th, 2008   03:48 pm

Carol Goad age 35, has breast cancer, and at present is beginning therapy at KU Med Center in KC Mo. She has 5 children from ages 8-16, a very lovely and caring mother. She is also in a trial for another cancer fighting drug which she will take for a year. They do not know what side effects she will have with this drug. She has Triple Negative Breast Cancer, a very aggressive fast growing cancer. Please give her encouragements..

Thursday, March 20th, 2008   03:26 pm

Carol has finished her first week of therapy; they are going to do therapy first and will do surgery after her chemo therapy is finished several months from now. It seems to be a new perspective on treatments. KU is top notch, high tech. A whole floor dedicated to Breast Cancer. We're very positive on every thing. She is also taking a pill a day to help the hospital learn (with the help of other ladies fighting this kind of cancer) about this unusual, aggressive form of cancer to see if it can be used in a helpful way in the future. They don't know what kind of side effects she may endure from this pill. She wants to help her children in the event they have this particular cell in the future.

. . . .

Upscale Treatment

The cancer center I went to was really very nice. Each person had their own cubical type room with a recliner, sink, DVD player, and your own nurse!

The first treatment took a little longer than the rest. They have to explain to you what happens in the event of an allergic reaction or in the event that the chemo was to spill or leak out under the skin and what to do. I remember thinking "Four hours for chemo? Really?" I mean it doesn't take that long to watch a movie, or cook dinner or clean the bathroom!

They do however have to give you all these pre-drugs in a series. I usually had a hard time lasting past administering the steroids and Benadryl. The first couple of times I was a little bit scared. I did not want to let these drugs "take me". I didn't want to lose control. I had no idea what the things were that they were giving me or how they were going to affect me. I was actually a little scared of something happening and not being able to articulate what I was feeling. I wanted to be awake the whole time so I knew what was going on. I remember sitting there fighting with everything in me to stay awake. My husband kept saying "Just relax babe, there are people here to take care of you." No matter how hard I fought I couldn't keep my eyes open.

At some point during the treatment I woke up and had to go to the bathroom. I thought "I can do this." I tried to stand up. My memory is fuzzy, but I know that I did try to make it to the door. My husband was trying to talk some sense into me. He was trying to help me. I didn't want help. I wanted to do it on my own. My husband said I ran into the door and was kind of stumbling. His exact words were "You were jacked up!" Bless his heart. I know it was hard to watch that and be pushed away. I laugh when I try to remember this because I do vaguely remember the nurse or my husband or heck who ever it was, asking me if I needed help once I got to the bathroom. I told them "No", that I was OK. What is funny though is when they shut the door and I attempted to "situate" myself, I realized that this could turn out to be very ugly and laughed at my predicament.

I wasn't really sure I could get myself back up and wash my hands so that I could make my way back to my little cubical. I just thought the last thing I want to have to holler out (and I know I really shouldn't make fun), is "Help!, I've fallen and I can't get back up!"

. . . .

Just
A
Little Bit

After a few days, with my husband and mom-in-law encouraging me to write what was going on to let all my family know, I sat down to write my first journal entry.

Friday, March 21, 2008   05:00 pm

Monday the 17th we went for what I thought was going to be my first chemo treatment, but found out that they have to give you steroids the day before to help with allergic reactions and what not. I had a CT scan and a MUGA scan. The MUGA scan I guess looks at your heart. This was all to get a baseline for how I look before and after therapy.

Tuesday the 18th I started chemo therapy. I signed the papers and was advised several times of the side effects, what was normal and what was not, and to call if there was anything at all that I needed. They put some pretty heavy stuff in my IV before starting the chemo so I slept through the majority of it. Travis and I stayed the night in KC with some close friends Monday night. I had more tests to do Wednesday but I was ready to see our kids and to be in my own bed so we went ahead and drove home. I think I slept a good majority of the ride home.

March 19th we drove back to KC. I had a bone scan and a Nulasta shot. The Nulasta shot brings my white blood cell count back up so that I can fight infection better. I am feeling tired and headachy but not bad at all.

March 20th. I'm feeling tired and a little yucky in the stomach. Other than the tummy ache my headache from yesterday is gone and I feel decent. Worried about what I can eat without paying the price. Went to town with my mom and picked up this water that my friend was telling me about. I hope to get some sleep tonight. I have not slept well the last two nights. But I did sleep decent last night! On the up side though, we have family and friends bringing dinner all week! WHAT A BLESSING that has been! Thank you! Thank you!

I can feel a little achiness in my knees today, but its nothing to really complain about. I am so so so thankful that so far it hasn't been too bad. My next appt. is April 7th. Travis and I will leave Sunday night because I have the first appt. in the morning. April 8th I will have the minor out patient surgery to have a port put in. Then three weeks until the next appt again!

I just want to tell you all that I am thankful for your prayers and thoughts. It is always fun to get a card in the mail as well! The kids love it, so I let them open the cards for me. I am trying to let Noah read them to me. At least the ones that aren't too difficult. It's good practice for him! In any case, Thank you!!!

By the way, I got my hair cut shorter today. I thought it might make things easier for me down the road. I can't wait to get my hands on some t-shirts that say LEAN MEAN CANCER FIGHTN MACHINE and start wearing them proudly! God and I, we've got major rump kicking to do!
Love you all, Carol

. . . .

Initially after my first treatment, I thought "Ok this isn't too bad." Then my knees started to ache. It was crazy. I remember wondering if that was how older people felt on a regular basis.

We went to the store the day after my chemo treatment. I was feeling a little off and my knees were starting to hurt but I wanted to keep up with my family and not loose any sense of normalcy. I wanted all this even though I felt physically like I was a little old lady. We got there and I was handling the knee thing ok. But we got about halfway through the store and I had a wave of exhaustion hit me like a ton of bricks. I seriously don't think I have ever felt so bone tired in my life. I didn't think I was going to make it to the front of the store. Now, I sit here and think about that, and I wonder how I really did make it to the front of the store.

The alternatives were running through my mind. I could send one of the kids to the front to get me an electric cart, but I am really *so* tired I don't even think I can operate the controls. The next option is I could climb into the cart, but where would they put the groceries? And the energy getting into the cart would be way more than I could muster. The last and most appealing option was to just lie in the floor at the end of the isle. I could just have one of the kids grab a leg and drag me from isle end to isle end. I didn't want any one to take me for dead or hurt though. They would end up calling the ambulance, lots of people would gather around, and well at this point I don't need that kind of attention.

So I settled for just perching on the end cap of stacked crackers. So if you bought a box of slightly smashed crackers from that end cap, I'm sorry, I really felt I had no other choice!

. . . .

Saturday, March 23rd, 2008 06:35 pm

Hi ya!

Well, today again is good! I am on my third day of trial drugs. I figured out if I take my nausea meds at the same time as the trial drug I feel pretty decent. I am also learning that by afternoon I am getting a little tired, so I need to plan accordingly.

We went to Nychelle's practice today. 3 ½ hours long! He must think that's all we have to do. Afterwards we grabbed a couple of soft tacos. I was starving so I decided I would endure what ever problems that might occur for eating it. Guess what? I am still alive and kicking! It didn't kick my rear! And I LOVE Mexican food!

Well I guess that's it!

Love Carol

. . . .

Easter was interesting. It was a little different in comparison to previous years. The reason is because my appetite was different. So the whole approach to family and food just felt different to me. I'm not sure how to describe it. I guess maybe I felt like something was missing.

I didn't have as much involvement as I have had before. Everyone else did the work for me. I had this constant stomach ache. Nothing would relieve it. Normally I would be a little frustrated by the second day of having a stomach ache. I think I came to a realization though that the way I was feeling was par–for-course and not nearly as tough as what I could be experiencing. I can tell you though that I have tried every flavor of antacids. The jury is still out on which flavor is my favorite. It usually depended on my mood.

. . . .

Tuesday, March 25th, 2008 08:07 am

Hey!

I hope everyone had a good Easter. We had dinner here at the house with my mom and step-dad, my step-mother and my father-in-law. It was nice. Everyone was making fun because I was eating a tiny bit of everything. The girls were calling it my sampler plate.
I'm learning what and how much I can tolerate. Later that evening we went to Travis' sisters house so that we could visit and see everyone for the holiday. That was nice as well.

Yesterday I felt horrible in the morning. I had what Travis is calling an anxiety attack. I have no idea. I called the Dr. just to be sure because I never felt any thing like that before and it was a little bit painful. I woke up yesterday with a sore tongue and sores in my mouth. I have been rinsing my mouth with baking soda several times a day in hopes that I wouldn't get these sores. Maybe it's at least keeping it at a tolerable level.

My face started breaking out something terrible too. Again I have been trying to take extra precaution in hopes that I would bypass that but, God has other plans I guess. I believe that we go through everything we do so that we can be sympathetic to others during their time of trial. If it makes me a better person, then I say bring it on. I understand that this next week I need to be a little extra careful as far as staying away from large crowds because of my blood count. I'm a little irritated with that as Nychelle has a tournament this weekend. I guess I can hope for a field that I can watch from a little ways back.

On the upside I've lost 6 pounds. Jell-O is my friend.

Well thanks for all the notes. They are very encouraging. I feel like superwoman with all the prayers going up! God has brought us to it, he will bring us through it!

Love you all

Carol

. . . .

When the sores started popping up in my mouth I thought "Oh crud, I *do not* want to deal with this." You know it's bad when you have nausea constantly, but adding little sores that are very irritating, can really test a person. There were times when I would stand in the bathroom at least five times a day, sometimes more, irrigating my mouth. I was looking for even the slightest amount of relief. I actually think it was the only time I had relief from those things.

About the same time my face started breaking out. I was taking an experimental drug that was in pill form. They put me on the highest dose. Well I had the side effect that was most common for that particular drug. My face was so raw and painful I couldn't really smile. I love to smile! My motto through those days became "It could be worse."

I always felt like I was a spiritual person, like God and I talked a lot, but maybe not like I do now. I think the way I learned to lean on God and put my faith and hope in him during this time, is what helped me get from minute to minute, day to day.

"Humble yourselves, therefore, under God's mighty hand, that he may lift you up in due time. Cast all your anxiety on him because he cares for you. –Resist him (the devil), standing firm in your faith, because you know that your brothers through out the world are undergoing the same kind of sufferings."

1 Peter 5:6,7,9

Sometimes you feel like no one else has a clue what *you're* going through. Like, yes, they have a similar situation but they haven't walked in *your* shoes. I felt like even though I was surrounded by all this love and people who wanted to help, I was sometimes alone. Not one person in my home *really* knew what is was like to walk out of the house with your face feeling and looking like it was on fire. But I pulled my chin up and I looked every one in the eye and I did what I needed to do to get through each day trying not to change much. I did that because I knew there is one person who knows our pain. There is one person who knows our heart. There is one person who knows when we are at our breaking point. When we put our faith in Him and we call out to Him, He extends His hand and pulls you from the floor to a standing position. He says through me, you can do all things. I placed my faith in Him that He would take care of this and my family. I have faith that He was trying to help me grow through this. So I tried to keep a great attitude, and I have tried to pay attention and understand what He has been trying to teach me. I now realize there was so much He was and is still trying to show me, that I have to keep a notebook and pen handy so I can put these pieces of the puzzle together.

I had this little red box of prayers that sat on our desk. At any time if I felt down at all, I would just pull one of them out.

"But seek first his kingdom and his righteousness, and all these things will be added to you"

Matthew 6:33

. . . .

Thursday, March 27, 2008 11:19 pm

Well, Hello my fluffy friends,

I guess I wrote in here Tuesday so I thought I would write again tonight.

With the exception of my face and mouth I actually felt normal today. If you saw my face right now you would be laughing.

I went to the dr. to see if she could give me anything for it. She did but I realized later that I have to stand on one foot, pat my head, rub my tummy, and jump back and forth through two hoops of fire so that I can actually HAVE the medication. Apparently the insurance company has to pre-approve the ointment. I seriously need a recorder so I can record the thoughts going through my mind about all of this. I crack myself up. Maybe if the recorder remembered it for me I could write it down later and as my cousin puts it, "make a gazabillion dollars off it and pay for some doctors nice ride".

So I go to pick up the meds at our local friendly large retailer. I am informed to call my prescription insurance company because the medication has to be pre-

approved. So I call, and they give me a dedicated line to pre-approvals. I go through the whole automated thing..... and it....can't understand... what drug...I'm spelling! Hold on. AHAHAHAHAHAHA! Seriously I am literally laughing out loud right now. Phew!

Ok, so, I wait for the live person, which sounds eerily like the automated girl. I give the information that I feel like I have already given 76 times! You won't believe this. She faxed the papers to my doctor right then and there, while I was on the phone with her. I know! Amazing! So I should have my medicine by the end of next week. By then maybe my face will be so swollen my eyes will be involuntarily shut. Maybe then I can take a really good picture so that maybe I can get some real sympathy.

Ok seriously all kidding aside, they tell me I should have it in a few days. Besides it cracks me up to see my family come home after they have been gone all day, and see their reaction. They apparently forget that I presently look like I have been drug down the road by my face by wild angry Ostriches. They actually wince when they see me. Nychelle teared up and Brice had to take a walk. Travis said "Babe, I'm glad you sound so good and are getting around good because when I first saw you I thought "Whoa!" Now imagine him pulling his head back and looking at you with big eyes as he says that. Again this tickled me. Apparently it DOES look worse than it feels. At that moment I was wishing I could have heard all the thoughts of the people at the store who dared look at me. Well maybe not. I would have been laughing so hard that I would have been in the floor peeing in my pants and they would have had to call maintenance to the pharmacy for clean up. And THAT would have only drawn more attention to my sad little condition.

Well thanks for the laugh. I have to go blow my nose now.....

Love Carol

I was not feeling well again, so my sweet mother-in-law wrote in my journal for me again.

Sunday, March 30th, 2008 8:38 pm

Just a few lines to bring Carol's journal up to date. She has been having a few days of not being up to par due to the trial medicine she presumes. We love her so much and hate to see her go through these extra problems. She is so chipper about everything. She will be back in a few days.

Shirley

Monday, March 31st, 2008 10:25 pm

Wasn't that sweet of my mom-in-law to write a line for me? I always tell her I struck gold when it comes to mother-in-laws!

Well the face thing the last few days has been very irritating. As I lay in bed last night in total torment my mind was racing. I was wondering if I should give it to you straight as far as the pain I was in or give it to you how it was running through my mind at the moment. The later version is more fun I think!

Who wants to read about normal run of the Joes pain anyhow…… but you'll like this.

So imagine this. Have you ever been in the shower and had it too hot? You know how you can bend over to pick up something or whatever and you get a little light headed?
Ok that was me last night. I thought to myself what would happen if I slipped right now? Everyone is in bed and here you are taking a shower. Would you call out? Or would you calmly lay there until you get the strength to pull yourself back up?

So I get this image in my head. I bend down to grab my razor, and I slip, and some how my foot becomes entangled in the string of the loofah sponge which happens to be hanging from the shower head. So here you are, this is what it comes down to. Somehow one leg is caught above your head in the loofah sponge and the other leg is somehow behind your head. What a predicament. I mean this is not a position you even want your husband to see you in. So I laugh imagining this, trying to come up with an escape plan in the event should this ever really occur.

The real fun happens after I get out of the shower. I decide to do my whole face regimen thing. This consists of very gently exfoliating all the dead skin from my face. After doing all this you can imagine the skin is somewhat raw and even mere lotion burns.

So I go through all my drawers looking for some thing to put on my face that won't burn. I spy antibiotic ointment. I have put this on some pretty deep cuts and never had it burn.

So I think PERFECT, it will SEAL and HEAL. So I am excited and busy slathering it on. So good so far. I proceed to take one contact out.....wait a MINUTE! It's burning...wholly moly......Burning! I'm thinking FOCUS Carol for the love of all that is good, FOCUS... get the other contact out. Finally I get the other contact out. Thank the Lord! Now all I can think is ICE! So I stumble half blind as quickly as possible to the fridge, all the while literally trembling in pain and trying not to cry out or laugh hysterically. I fill up a zip lock bag with crushed ice. I then move quickly back to my bathroom for a wet wash cloth and head to bed. Then I remember CRUD! I didn't take the Benadryl.

As I have told you all before, this is to help offset allergic reactions and right now I'm just hoping it will help me get to sleep quicker. So I pull out the little suckers that are at this point, as far as I'm concerned, sealed in military wrapping. For the love of Horney toads! It's just Benadryl! I can't get the wrapping off! In the mean time my face feels like acid is covering it. The ice is sitting on the counter tormenting me. FINALLY I manage to get the drug opened and down my throat. I move to the bed, now feeling a bit on the side of loony crazy and lay down.

I put the ice across my face. AHHHH! The ice is my friend. I turn it and turn it and pray for the Benadryl to kick in so that I can fall asleep. As I realize I'm going to live, I thank God for ice and automatic ice crushers, plastic bags and the fact that my husband neither had to rescue me out of the shower or call 911. All in all is been a pretty good day.

I woke up this morning and my face looked pretty darn good. Who says beauty doesn't hurt? My KU doctor. prescribed a new med for this little problem today. I can already see it's working. I'm SUCH a moron! Why didn't I call him last week? The insurance denied approval on the ointment. Well, phewy, I'm sure that ointment doesn't have anything on good ol' Neosporin!

So maybe in the next few days I will look normal again. I think I have convinced Travis that I can actually drive now. I CAN still drive! Give me freedom!

Well love you guys, one more week and it's controlled poison day! Yeah!

Carol

Monday, March 31st, 2008 11:14 pm

Oh hey one more thing, I just want to thank you guys who are all writing in the guest book. I so look forward to reading them.

I really feel like you are all my personal angels God has assigned me. And through you, sometimes I hear him whisper. I need all of your words of encouragement. I just wanted you to know that.

Love you
C

. . . .

You know that night was crazy. I remember *really* feeling like I was shy of loony. The pain was so intense. What I wanted to do was lay my face in the bucket of the ice dispenser. I *can not* explain to you the relief I felt when I put that ice pack on my face.

When I laid down, I was on the brink of tears, but within a few minutes I just felt like laughing. I am going to live to see yet another day!

. . . .

Wednesday, April 2, 2008   11:03 am

Travis walked in yesterday, and when I saw his face the flood gates opened. Sometimes you just want space to breath, to feel normal. I haven't had that in a few weeks except for what I create in my own demented little mind.

I had three people last week, out of the blue just call or tell me I was beautiful. One was Travis, one was my sister, and one was one of my daughter's friends, who is like one of my own. Now normally I would say something cute and light hearted like "Your right, and aren't you lucky to be on the receiving end." But when you are walking around with nastiness all over your face, and hey, let's face it, that's what people notice first, beautiful is not in the vocabulary. So each time those people said that to me, I felt blessed that somehow they knew just what my heart needed to hear.

Now most who know me personally, know that I am not by any means vain. I do not usually wear makeup. But I'm here to tell you that when this is all over with, I am going to slather it on. I'm going to try every color available! Tammy Faye will have nothing on me! I am going to buy false eye lashes in every color and with every possible sparkle in it!

How's the rash? Well it's going great, it's keep'n on keep'n on. We will figure out the brains of the operation and shut it down soon, I have no doubt!

My girls are having a hat party for me this week end. It sounds like fun.

Well that's it for today I guess,

Love Carol

Wednesday April 4th, 2008 6:26 pm

Hello!

You know what I'm listening to right now? Love is a battlefield. I think that is Pat Benatar right? Isn't that true? Love IS a battlefield. But so is life.

Well, we are going to the lake this evening. I haven't been there in a while. I am excited to go say hello to the lake and hear the ducks! We will be coming back sometime Saturday though. This is so we can get our stuff together to head to K.C. Sunday afternoon. Monday I get to see my Doc, get my blood checked, and then go do the wonderful chemo. It's not so bad because they give me this stuff that makes me feel all warm and fuzzy. I sleep.

So Travis is bored to death for a few hours. We will bring him a movie this time though. Then on Tuesday we will get up and get to the hospital by 6:30 am so I can have the port put in. I guess I will have just enough time to recover before we leave for the hospital and head back over to the cancer center for an MRI. Then back upstairs to have the Nulasta shot and then home!

So that is what we are doing for the next few days.

Anyhoo, when we go to the lake, we get bacon for breakfast, so we are all very excited! It is quite the treat for us. Since Travis had his heart attack, we just don't keep the stuff around. So if you happen to invite us for breakfast and you cook bacon, please don't torture us by allowing only two little strips of bacon a piece. Buy the pig and we will love you forever!

Bacon is our friend!

Love you all

Carol

The poem on the next page is how I feel most of the time. My dad always said "Just another day in paradise", long before Phil Vassar ever sang it.

It's truly how he dealt with the good and bad. The fact is, life is what we make it. I won't sit here and pretend I don't feel weighted sometimes but, I knew something my dad was just starting to think about.

I know a wonderful and powerful God who has a plan for me. I just have to surrender in faith that he will put me where I need to be. Sometimes that means going through trials in our lives.

Thank you Tosh, for sending this to me.

This Too Shall Pass

I can endure this minute
Whatever is happening to me,
No matter how heavy my heart is
Or how dark the moment may be-

If I can remain calm and quiet
With all the world crashing about me,
Secure in the knowledge God loves me,
When everyone else seems to doubt me.

If I can but keep on believing
What I know in my heart to be true,
That darkness will fade with the morning
And that this will pass away, too-

Then nothing in life can defeat me

For as long as this knowledge remains

I can suffer whatever is happening

For I know God will break all the chains

That are binding me tight in the darkness

And trying to fill me with fear-

For there is no night without dawning

And I know that my morning is near.

H. Rice

This poem was one of my favorites.

I go back and read it from time to time. At the time, the last two lines packed a punch for me. “For there is no night without dawning, and I know that my morning is near.”

You know there is no dawn without God.

No dawn without God, no night without dawn and morning is near. For every bottom there is a top. For every door that closes one opens. Life goes on. This is true even if you pass away. Your loved ones have to go on living.

God has a purpose for every single person he put here.
While you’re here, grasp what it is your supposed to be doing.

Your morning is near.

This is another entry from my mother-in-law.

Tuesday, April 8, 2008   01:35 pm

Carol had treatment yesterday. They are now on their way home. In a few days the effects of the chemo will hit her and she may not be up to par. I know she will write as soon as she can.

. . . .

It is about a two and a half hour trip from our home to KC. There is a lot of time to talk, and well, get anxious.

You know, chemo can make you cold from the inside out. Sometimes it was actually painful. I'm not talking about while they are giving you the chemo. I'm talking about what it does hours and days after it's in you.

There were nights I was so cold I was in pain and shaking. I had extra comforters folded in half on my side of the bed. I would also lie on a heating pad. One night in particular I remember laying there, trying hard not to chatter my teeth. I began thinking, "If this is what hypothermia feels like, then No Thank You!" This will be added to the things I definitely don't want to die from.

. . . .

Wednesday, April 9, 2008   8:23 pm

This is Travis. I'm going to throw in the word before Carol gets started with her crazy writings!

Mark 14:30 starts to explain how the lord reveals that tonight, before the rooster crows twice, Peter will disown him three times. Peter was insistent that this was not the case. The Lord is amazing, he loves us, he knows we will betray him, and yet he still loves us! He is calling out to Peter and he still loves him. I can only imagine how Peter felt when Christ returned and called his name.

This story reminds me personally that Christ loves us like a mother and father loves their children. It does not matter what the case, if we turn our backs, do/say/or even think the wrong idea about life or Christ himself, he is still there, loving us, waiting for us to return to him, wrapping us in his arms and warming our hearts with love. Sometimes I wonder why, why, why, and I start to doubt, and continue to use my small brain to try and figure it all out, but no matter what, we have to keep our faith and know the Lord is just around the corner and he will pick us up and lift us higher than we could ever imagine.

Wednesday, April 9, 2008 8:23pm

What you don't know is how Travis and I were feeling coming home yesterday. It felt like the weight of the world was on our shoulders. It's amazing how a few prayers, some talking and a nights rest can change your perception of what is really going on in your life.

So after reading what Travis just wrote I thought I should let you know that although for the most part we try to keep our heads up, sometimes doubt rushes in.

Sunday we left for K.C. and had to be there by 6 am to check into what they call the Hope Lodge. It's free lodging for cancer patients that is in downtown K.C. It was a really nice place. The people there are super and treated us like family.

Monday we had to be at the cancer center by 8 am for blood work, to see the doctor and then chemo. They said my blood work looked great and that I didn't need another Nulasta shot. My Dr. was very excited that we sent him pictures. He is foreign and I love to hear his accent. I am smiling the whole time we are there talking. Then he says "but your face was so so sad in those pictures." I then told him that my dang face and lips were so swollen, that if somebody did make me smile, it would of hurt! He said "Well we will take care of that."

Travis and I get to cracking up pretty good if they leave us in the room too long. I'm sure they wonder what we are up to. My hair is coming out pretty good now. Travis asked me to pull a few strands of my hair out while we are sitting there to see how easily it came out. Well, he freaked out and decided he needed to pull on some himself too. He says "Oh my gosh, Carol!" Then he says you know what you should do, it is coming out so easily that you should wait till we get home and the girls start arguing, then grab a bunch of hair on each side of your head and pull. That would startle them for sure!
He said you could tell them "Look what you're doing! You're literally causing me to pull my hair out!"

We had a good laugh over that.

You want to hear something hilarious? I'm gonna tell on myself.

Sunday it was a little windy. We were at the girl's ball practice before we left out, so my hair had been flappin in the wind for a little while. With Travis behind the wheel, we start on our way to K.C. I start finger combing my hair to get it smoothed out. Well as I mentioned earlier the stuff is jumping ship on me, so with each swipe I have hair coming out. With my right hand I roll down the window to throw the hair out, with my left hand I attempt to throw the wayward hair out the window. With no warning WHATSOEVER, my right hand gets sneaky and rolls the window up on my left hand! My thumb is screaming! I panic and start yelling OW! OW! OW!

I look over my left shoulder at Travis with I'm sure some measure of desperation and wanting him to help. Like the wonderful husband he is, he slaps himself on the forehead and with a smile and says "Roll the window down!" Ahhh! Why didn't I think of that? Somehow my brain engages and tells my right hand to have mercy on my left hand and push the window button. My left thumb is quite sore and is still not fully cooperating with any of my right hands doings at this time.

Tuesday I had the port put in. It was kind of weird because they didn't put me all the way under. I could hear them talking, and the radio playing during the surgery. But I didn't feel anything and that's really the important part anyway isn't it?

After having the port put in we went straight back over to the cancer center for the MRI. Now when you have an MRI on your breast it's kind of strange. Basically they have these two holes you dangle your "girls" through so they can take pictures. I'm thinking, seriously? This can't be done on my back? The crazy thing is they say "here are some ear plugs, take off your gown, crawl..... yes crawl up there and put your girls in those holes, stretch your arms above your head, and if you hear clicking noises that sound as if something could slice them off, not to worry, you'll be OK!" Somehow through all the clicking and whirring (why is that thing so loud anyway), I did actually take a nap. I'm sure that was due to the 1000 mg of Hydrocodone they gave me after surgery so I wouldn't be in too much pain lying on my newly installed port.

Holy cow, I'm writing a book. So I will wrap it up. My stomach is killing me anyhow. I feel ok for the most part, except that everything taste like crud, my stomach hurts and my shoulder hurts. It could be worse they say. I could be in the bathroom 24/7. This probably wouldn't be too awful of a place. It gets visited a lot and I do have four girls, so the chance of getting my hair done would be a lot better if I hung out in there more!

Well TaTa for now!
Love you all
Carol

. . . .

The hair I was losing was getting irritating. I told Travis I felt like a cat. Every time someone picked me up, I left a ton of hair behind. It was beginning to get a little nutty.

At some point in April there was discussion in my house about when to go ahead and get my head shaved. I decided to call a friend of mine and she got me in that day. Although it was a little emotional for me that day, I think it was more surreal than anything. All of my girls, one of their friends, Alisha, and one of the other girls in the shop (Ellen) were so sweet and gentle. I appreciated them so much! My Husband was sweet as well. He kept asking me if I was ok. I just kept smiling and saying "Yes babe, don't worry."

It was weird.... Shaving your head is weird. I looked in the mirror. Someone vaguely familiar stared back. Weird. Looking back now I wish I would have just tried all different kinds of wigs. I think to myself now, "Self? If you had it to do again would you have changed much?" My answer? "Nope, probably not"

. . . .

Tuesday, April 15th, 2008 12:47pm

Hi there,

Just so you know this is the second time writing this. I lost it the first time which was yesterday. It was a little frustrating to say the least.

I'm not sure what to write about. There must be something, it's been a week.

Curser blinking.

Wednesday and Thursdays were not good days. Friday was better and so on and so forth. Friday I learned not to take one of my pills with the morning pills. BAD idea.

I also learned Saturday morning that a bald head makes 39 degree weather feel a WHOLE LOT colder.

More later-----

Thursday, April 17th, 2008 09:24pm

Well hello my friends and family,
I have had some serious issues getting on here and writing something this week. I don't know why.

Well I guess I will start with the hat party the girls threw for me. It was standing room only and much fun! I received moose hats, chicken hats, every possible variation of pink hat, sun hats, cool hats, collector hats, scarfs and do-rags. In addition I scored flip flops, tea, words of wisdom, and cards.

People brought cake and food. I think everyone had a good time! I have over 87 hats at last count I think. Enough that I could wear one every day and not get bored for quite a while! My daughters and their friend hustled restaurants and got free gift certificates to give away as well as some candle sets and pillows as party gifts. They had one of the local grocery stores give them $50 to spend as they pleased for the things for the party as well. They wanted to do this on their own. And they did a great job. I'm very proud of them!

I have to tell you, we were exhausted Saturday night. When I got my head shaved one of my daughters friends wanted so very badly to shave her head to show her love and support for me. But I threatened her and told her absolutely not. Well later that night my step sister left and came back.

When I saw her my jaw dropped!

She went and had her head shaved. (She had obviously forgotten to take her medication.) I was floored. And I'm not gonna lie, a little upset. I didn't WANT to shave my head. Why would she do that?!?! She said "I didn't want you to feel alone." I love her, but that was just plain crazy!

This week has been decent as far as how I have been feeling. I did have all the regular run of the mill stuff. In the afternoons I'm tired but all in all nothing major to complain about. I have however been having pain in my arm since Thursday or so of last week. I just kept thinking I hadn't healed up yet from having the port put in. Well, I have been wearing long sleeve shirts all the time because I'm always freezing. So I hadn't really noticed any swelling. I noticed yesterday while I was getting dressed that my arm was swollen and had this raised red band around it.

So I checked my paper work then got online to research it. I then called my doc at K.U. and then called Travis. He came home got me and took me to St. Johns. Long story short they found a blood clot in my arm that they think might be either from the last I.V. I had or a slim chance from the port. It was in a superficial vein, one that is close to the skin. So they sent me home and advised me to put heat on it and take an anti-inflammatory. So far it seems to be helping and I am SO glad.

Softball is in full swing so it is something every night. I don't mind it though, really.
My sister is doing a poker run Saturday if anyone is interested, and a friend of mine is putting together a benefit at the High school in May.

Today my mom took me running around town and we had lunch like big people. That was fun. She will be here till tomorrow I think.

Well peeps I guess that's it for now. I'm still alive and kicking! The other day my oldest daughter was upset about my hair and that I have to go through all this. But I explained to her that it really was ok, and that it was a means to an end. I will gladly give up my hair for life. Seems like a real fair trade for me.

I'm obviously bald now. It just seemed wrong to lint roller myself 17 times a day. AND I wasn't getting near the attention anymore so I had to up the anti and shave it off. Now that *shock is starting to wear off...You think flames tattooed across the side of my head will do it? We will see!*

Love you all   C

. . . .

My mom stayed with us while I was sick and sort of set up camp at our house. My sister would come by sometimes and my mother-in-law came out and helped too. My mom was here a lot though. She did laundry, picked up things at the store, cleaned and so many other things. I really appreciate her for that. I also appreciate my step-dad, as he did without her all those days and nights she was here with me.

When extended family comes in, camps out and helps it is difficult. This is something that gets talked about very little as well. Cancer is disruptive in itself but, when someone else comes in and tries to help, sometimes just those sweet people trying to help is disruptive. It's just the nature of the beast. In each of our households we have our own system of how things are run. So when you step into someone else's house, we end up doing things our own way. When our own way does not line up with the already established system of the house things can get a little hairy. This is a kind of what happened in our house.

She kept everything running, in order, and in good shape for the most part. The kids were pretty good for the most part as well. I do think they tested my mom a few times. I think they decided they didn't like her a few times, as she decided to "learn them" in areas I didn't have the energy to. It was probably good for her! I do think I have great kids though. So I'm pretty sure it wasn't as bad as it probably could have been.

You see I am also a stay at home mom. So I carry the burdon of most the chores in the house. I am a fairly laid back mom, so sometimes just half way getting something done is ok with me. I mean, I am appreciative of the half way work... because, you know, there could be no work at all! My mom on the other hand, does not operate like that.

Let me elucidate.

When I was a kid, my chore was the kitchen. She tried to "train" me to believe that cleaning the stove was part of doing the dishes. Now I did do that part of the job when I lived at home. But when I moved out I rebelled and decided to only clean the stove if someone special was coming over. (Believe me, there are very few people who are THAT special!). Do you see where I'm going with this? So there is MY mom in MY kitchen, with rebellion all over the stove. Bless her heart. She did good though. So I guess if you're helping or being helped, know that it is going to be disruptive and try to defuse any situation as soon as it arises.

. . . .

Friday, April 18, 2008 03:14am

Do not pay attention to the time of the post. It was held in queue too long, or it could be a figment of your imagination.

I can't sleep. I tried. I even tried counting sheep backwards but I kept getting the giggles because they kept tripping over the fence.

I didn't want to wake Travis up. So I got outta bed and came in here to try and find some other TNBC (Triple Negative Breast Cancer) people. And then found myself back here.

I must have woke mom up. She just stopped by to say hello.

I was laying there thinking that the next time I get on here I'm gonna thank all those cool people for telling me to be strong, and that I am strong and what not. You know my first reaction is to roll my eyes like a teenager and say "whatevah." Then my next reaction is to say "GEE Gorsh", you know, like Goofy. (Is he a dog?) Then my final reaction is to roll up my shirt sleeve, show my muscle, pop the can of spinach out of my back pocket and throw that green stuff to the back of my throat. I would swallow just in time to look over and watch all my muscles pop just like Popeye. After he has eaten all the spinach, you know he's invincible then? So I guess my point is, when you say those things I go through all those emotions and finally end on something that ultimately sustains me. Thank you for that.

Talking about Popeye always makes me think of my dad. I know you get on here to get an update about me, but do you mind if I talk about him for a sec? My dad was a real life Popeye. He was built like him too. My dad unexpectedly passed away November 2.

I don't talk about him a whole lot for that cements that he is really gone. He is a good part of why I am who I am, and why I look at life like I do. I talked to him late afternoon the day before he died. He called to tell me Happy Birthday. He called and joked and we laughed as usual. But the unusual thing that I will always remember is that he must have told me at least 4 times in that short phone call that he loved me. I mean he always told me he loved me, but he kept saying it over and over again. I remember laughing and saying yes dad I know you do, I love you too.

You see my dad was not just any old dad, he was amazing. What I'm about to tell you Travis' family knows but some of mine don't. Do you know when Travis had his heart attack my dad took a week off of work to be by his side without pay? He never left. He loved Travis that much. He couldn't afford to do that but he did.
He used to say "It's just another day in paradise" long before it was a song. He smiled the biggest goofiest smile he could muster. I told him one time that the next time he saw me, if he was gonna tell me jokes it had to be clean.

I told him some of the other jokes were terrible and not good for my kid's ears. So sure enough the next time I see him, he grabs me by my arm and says "Carol Anne, Carol Anne! I got a joke for ya!" so I roll my eyes and say "OOOK?" He said "No you will like this one. What did the snail say when the turtle gave it a ride?" I give him an uncertain smile and said "I don't know dad, what?" He said "WHEEEEEEEE!", in this high pitched squeal.. I laughed. I gave him a hug and told him thank you. That was years ago, whenever I can, I tell that joke.

So I guess I'm just trying to say I miss my dad something terrible right now. He always promised me he would outlive me. You know I believed him. God had other plans.

Well thanks for letting me vent, maybe I can go in there and get some sleep now.

Night, or rather... Morning

With love
Carol

Saturday, April 19, 2008   09:24pm

Hey guys,

Well, the poker run that my sister set up today was interesting. I decided after hanging out and seeing all the people in and out of the Harley store, that I believe I want to be a biker chick. Right after my son goes off to college anyway. I want to be a full on biker chick though. I want the cool bike with the ghost flames and all the leathers and boots and stuff. I have the fever!

For the record I did finally get to sleep the other night in case you were losing sleep worrying about it. My arm is feeling better. I am almost at the end of my Tarceva run for this treatment and my face still looks good.

(It started healing up about 2 ½ weeks ago.) I guess the lower dosage and other drugs have helped keep it at bay. I've only been taking one of those extra pills instead of two this whole time. I'm not thrilled about taking all these pills so where ever I can fudge and it not hurt me I will. Well it has been a long full day. I watched my nephew play ball this evening. I love it. Now I need to go sit on the couch and pass out while watching t.v. so I can go to bed and actually sleep. Lame I know, but so true.

I am anxious to hear from you so I'll be waiting on pins and needles.... Ok or just the couch

Love you all!
Carol

. . . .

I was thinking how thankful I am that my doctors saw fit to put me through chemo first then surgery.
When they say breast conserving surgery, that's exactly what happened for me. I was really worried about that part. Not because I'm vain but because emotionally it's a big deal.

I have a little bit of advice for those who have not personally went through breast cancer. The last thing you should say is "Only society puts importance on breasts, you can get reconstructive surgery if you want." "They have those inserts and special bra's so no one will ever know."

But I know. It's a process. These things take time.

Luckily I did not have to go through that. The chemo shrunk my tumor. When they did surgery they only had to remove a small amount of breast tissue. By looking at my breast now, you can only tell by two small scars that there was an issue.

I am blessed. I am thankful.

. . . .

Friday, May 02, 2008   12:33pm

Hello all my lovely's,

All I have been praying for is warm sunny weather. When I do get it, it's all I can do to keep my eyes open.

I know it has been awhile. My 3rd week I tend to try to really do a lot because after treatment I know I'm toast.

Then of course I had treatment Monday. I did get some good news though. The tumor is shrinking! They put a plastic marker in the middle because they say some times the tumor shrinks so much all they can find is the marker! That's what I'm hoping for, nuthin but marker!

The actual treatment went a lot smoother this time. They were able to access my port and all went well there. I have had some pretty good fatigue this time. Today seems to be better though. I feel like I have totally missed the entire week. I did get to watch my son play ball though. It was nice to be outside in the fresh air. I sat there on the benches thinking, "If these people wouldn't think I was weird, I would lay down right here and watch this game." Even though I was tired I really felt a sense of peace, and maybe even well-being. Life is so short and we get so busy and caught up, sitting still and feeling the breeze is the last thing we think about.

On Monday I had another biopsy. It will tell them more about the trial drug I have been taking. The MRI did not show any other cancer, so that was good news as well.

I was telling my sister the other day that I was getting a little uncomfortable for how enthusiastic the Dr. was for taking core samples from my tumor. I mean I heard the nurse say we only needed three. Well he took those three then said, "So why don't we get one more while I am here?" They say ok. He says again, "You want another one?" The girls say "No I think we are good." The Dr. says "One more for the road." He then proceeds to ask me if it hurts. I say "On the inside or outside?" The answer is yes and no."

Let me tell you about this little procedure. They have you get undressed in a fairly warm room, put on a little throw thing and move you to a meat locker. After you have chilled for just about the right amount of time, they take you down a long white hall way. If you're not paying very close attention here you could get lost. They then take you into a room with a tiny table that looks like its hiked up to the ceiling. You then get on the table and expose your breast. Now if that's not enough, they have to roll you to your side and slide this wedge thing underneath your shoulder blade. Now if there is ever a time that you want someone to see you displayed like this, now is it! I mean that wedge took at least 10 years off my breast! I was hollering out the door, "Come on in, the waters fine!" just praying all the cute docs in the facility would hear me. Seriously, if you're ever going to take a picture of your breast, (and we don't know why) lay down, stuff a wedge under your breast, and vwaa laaa, instant beautiful breast!

Talk to you soon
Love you all!
Carol

. . . .

I felt like I was going along just fine. Doin' my thing. You know, your self-sufficient, helping others when you can, then all of a sudden something runs out right in front of you. You have to put on the brakes and reassess the situation.

It's hard to accept help when you are the one who is usually giving the help. So many people from our community wanted to help us. It was humbling. We had to learn to switch our attitude of "No thank you, we are doing ok." to "Wow, thank you so much that would be so great or so helpful."

A man's pride will bring him low,
But a humble spirit will obtain honor
Proverbs 29:23

I think all these people were just a way for God to show us he loved us. That he knows at some points in our lives, we feel discouraged, and therefore he sends people to cross our paths who will encourage us.

In his kindness God called you to share in his eternal glory
by means of Christ Jesus.
So after you have suffered a little while,
he will restore, support, and strengthen you,
and he will place you on a firm foundation.
1 Peter 5:10

. . . .

Monday, May 5th, 2008   10:03 AM

You know, I'm not a preachy kind of person.
I like to see living examples of God, not someone telling me how I should be living.

This is exactly what led me into a personal relationship with God as an adult. (Let me just clarify, I always knew God, felt like he was in my life, but maybe I wasn't living through or for him like I should.)

I witnessed two people who were living a life like I wanted. I'm not talking about stuff. Actually one of these people struggled financially and the other was, well she was blessed and had what she needed. I'm talking about a glow that surrounded them. I'm talking about people who also were not preachy, but they didn't have to be. You could feel it. They had a trust in God like nothing I had ever seen. (And actually until I learned to understand it, I thought a few times they were right close to crazyville.) Every time you are in their presence there is just warmth and a real peace. I don't want to embarrass the one who reads this so I won't say his name. The other one has taken her ride to heaven already. Now that's not to say that I don't know tons of people who are amazing Godly people as I think that most the people who are close to us are. But at this particular point in my life I believe I have seen something that I'm not real sure I've ever had my eyes opened to before.

Why am I telling you this? I don't know. I think because I want you all to know I'm OK. That I take this on as a challenge that God has lent my family because he knew we could endure it to learn from it. I am trying to be a different person every day. I am finding I have a passion for things that maybe I was scared of before. But I welcome it, whatever it may be. (Ok except for maybe the vomiting part, hey I know that's gross, but seriously that makes me cry) So please keep praying for me because I know God is hearing you and answering prayers. But know that emotionally and really even physically I am doing OK.

~So, Saturday was good. They apparently sold a lot of hotdogs. I guess they were good because I heard people were buying 2 and 3 hotdogs and leaving the chips behind. The music was amazing as well. There was some awesome stuff up there and some deals to be had, so if you didn't come, you missed out!

We were all talking about become professional benefit hoppers. We could get all of our Christmas shopping done at fantastic prices! The eats are generally cheap too! AND you are helping someone! Where else can you go to get your Christmas shopping done, enjoy entertainment (usually), and eat while helping a family? I'm seriously going to start doing that! It's an easy inexpensive way to feed the family, get out of the house and did I mention your HELPING someone? Hey, maybe we could all do it together. We could form a benefit hopping club or something. We can meet up once a month and help someone. So, if you are game, think of a cool name we can call this club. I really don't think it is gonna work without a cool name.

I am so appreciative of everyone who has shown us so much love. My heart aches. I really want to do something for all these people to show them how much I truly appreciate everything. I pray God blesses them tenfold in the very near future, but dang it, I wanna do something too!

Well, I suppose I'm done talking now. I thank you guys again for writing in here. You have no idea how some days it lifts me up.

I love you all
C

. . . .

I should probably save this little bit of information for my next book, but I have to share this.
I used to tell my kids when I had one-on-one time with them that they were my favorite. I would tell them the things I loved about them and tell them it was really important for them not to tell their sisters or brother as we didn't want to hurt their feelings. I would explain to them that their heart would be broken so it was important to keep this just

between us. (I did this with secret ice cream cones too for awhile, hahaha.)

After/During chemo I was walking around in a drug induced stupor half the time. What I'm trying to say is, I got sloppy. I started telling them they were my favorite when others were around. Needless to say, I got caught. One child heard me say this to another in one of my sloppy moments. That child said "HEY! You said I was your favorite!" So, as I'm sure you can imagine, I had to do some pretty quick dancing.

The word got out to the other kids, and well I sort of felt bad. How I found out, was one day I told my middle child (my favorite hehehe) that, well, you know, that I loved her and that she was my favorite.
She then said, in maybe not so many words, "Drop the act mom. We all know what's going on. We know you have been telling ALL of us that!" (I'm fairly certain there was a bit of eye rolling in there as well) I feigned surprise and disgust at the mere thought that she would suggest something like that. She just gave me a smile and with rolled eyes (once again) "Whatever Mom."

So now I tell them that they are all my favorite, but make sure to add their name in front of it. For example, "Alex, do you know you're my favorite daughter named Alex?" Eyes rolling. Alex quips with a smile, "Wow thanks Mom, I feel special, since I'm your ONLY daughter named Alex." I respond "SO? That should make it EXTRA special". Again, eye rolling. "Ok, Mom."

I hope my kids know I love all of them with all I have.

(AND that they are ALL my individual favorites!)

I know that had absolutely nothing to do with cancer. I just like that story.

. . . .

Saturday, May 24, 2008 7:13 am

Hey guys!

I know it's been a little bit since I have written. But in the famous words of my children, "It's not my fault!", or wait, maybe it's "I didn't do nuthin!" Either way I have some catching up to do. It may take a couple of days to accomplish that though, because there is a lot to tell.

My hubby got on here about a week and a half ago or so and said "Carol have you been on the Caringbridge site?" I said "No, something is wrong with my PC." "Hhmmm" was his response. A few days later he asked me to get on the computer and check something for him. I said, "I would love to do that but there is something wrong with the PC."

We are on our way to treatment on Monday, and he asked me "Hey have you been in on your site in a while?" I look at him as if he has lost his mind. I speak very slowly with a slight grin. Not too much teeth. You know, I don't want to start an argument here. I say, "Travis, you remember when I told you I was having problems with my computer and I couldn't blah blah blah? Yeah Ok, well, I can't do much but surf the web at this point, SO when you get a chance you might want to *take a look at it." Travis says "Oh." This was Monday. Three days later, on Wednesday we are getting ready to go to the lake. This is our ritual. Cancer or not, in sickness and in health, it matters not whether we have $50 or $500, we head to the great waters of Oklahoma. It is our family sanity time. All ball stops, heck all the world could stop. Really, seriously, come rain, storms, or sunshine that is where we set up home every Memorial weekend. As a matter of a fact I am writing this to you while sitting inside listening to the rain and wind, praying that the current storm does no damage and everyone comes out of their tents semi dry.*

Now back to my story. Travis asks me Wednesday morning, "Hey babe did you register Brice for Softball?" I walk into the living room, making sure I make eye contact with him and say, "I – Can – Not – Use – My – Computer – For – Such - Things my lovely honey pumpkin bunches of dumplings. I have tried to explain this to you several times." Now, I know this sounds crazy, like I'm making all this up, but seriously it was as if lightning struck right then and there in our living room. I witnessed a miracle! Travis then said, "OH! I will go take a look at that!" HOLY MOLY! You're kidding? I'm thinking, should I offer the guy a drink? Maybe he could use a freshly fluffed pillow? A scalp massage while he works? Hey, WHATEVER it takes! He is MOVING TOWARDS THE COMPUTER!

I'm just teasing you guys. He takes care of stuff

So we get down here (to the lake). He drags his little lap top computer out. He then says "Man babe you really haven't done anything on here." (Meaning Caringbridge) Ok, Pop Quiz. Have you been following along closely? Are you sure? Why haven't I been able to write on Caringbridge? Let's make this fun. The first person to write in with the correct answer gets a free set of steak knives. (I know I have some out in the barn somewhere) Please allow 8 to 12 weeks for delivery. (I have to find them ok?)

By the way, to his credit, Travis did fix the computer, but we left right after that so I didn't get a chance to write.

So, finally, here I am. I'm going to try to fill you in a bit. I feel decent this week as far as those things go. I was telling my friend that I think some of my issues are self-induced. For instance I have this terrible taste in my mouth all the time. It gets a little better the closer it gets to treatment each time. But after each treatment it's terrible. When I eat or drink something it seems to make it worse. So then if I even think about eating or drinking, in my head I get all sick and then eventually think I'm going to get physically sick. It's a vicious cycle. I am trying to reprogram myself in that area and see if I can change that. On the up side, I keep losing weight. I told Travis that if I lost 20 more pounds, I just might be ready to go under the knife. I hear that they now do a thing where they take fat and a piece of muscle to help with breast reconstruction. "So?" You say? Well, my friends that basically means a small over haul! We are talking about a new boob AND a tummy tuck! Who says cancer doesn't have its kickbacks! I have to tell you, I relayed this incredible information to my oldest. She looked at me as if I were an alien. I live for those moments.

I'm going to change gears a little bit here. We lost Aunt Lola, and recently another family friend "Bob". I feel the need to discuss certain things in light of these losses. For instance, I should probably let people know where I keep things. Seriously, when someone you love passes, and they don't have the luxury to tell you how they want things done, and maybe where certain things are at, it can be time consuming and on occasion frustrating. I know when my dad passed I wish we would have gotten 3 free calls to ask him a few things. Unfortunately, life just doesn't work like that.

Also, I wanted to make sure that everyone knew what I wanted a head of time. We get a little irrational in our grieving process sometimes don't we? So, I'm gonna make it easy on you all. It's right here in black and white. Don't worry my hats are up for grabs, so it's first come first serve! Moving on to the important stuff. My funeral should be light hearted. Everyone please just wear jeans and tennis shoes, or whatever you woke up in. (Please don't forget to brush your teeth, this is for the comfort of everyone around you) I would like a "Wake". This is just in case I actually decide to do just that. If I am too tired or too far gone to "Wake", then just put me in whatever is affordable. My dad always said to just put him out in the trash can. As lovely and comfy as a trash can sounds, I'm sorry, but I have to draw the line there.

As I have already discussed with some family members, you would have to get a person in a trash can pretty quick after death if that's what you so choose. Bodies are only pliable for so long. I am fairly sure mine will be no different. I don't want to cause any undue stress as far as trying to get me to the can in time........ hahahahahahahahaha. Ok that was just wrong, but funny.

I will require many people to congregate, and eat food for however many days it will take to keep my family sane. I don't care what kind of band you hire as long as everyone is sort of having a good time. Travis will need to be heavily medicated, so trust me, he won't care either. Or, hey, you could just hire a D.J. and all bring your own cd's! You should also feel free to dance and mingle or even get a softball game going. That would fantastic!

So we are clear, I love you all equally. You are all my favorite! Ok!
Well, the rain has stopped. I will write again soon. I have so much to tell.
Love you all Carol

. . . .

Somewhere between my last post in May, and my next post in June, I must have been busy. I know we must have had ball games and all the things that keeps our summers busy. I do remember those last treatments getting a little rough. I

started dry heaving, feeling sick longer, and just having a hard time lifting my head off the pillow for very long lengths of time. I didn't want to be in bed all the time though because I didn't want my kids to feel weird about what was going on with me. I have had several discussions with my family and people who were around me during my treatment. I thought I was in bed very little. Everyone else seems to think I was always laying down. Well, I say that I had the SPIRIT of being up! Whether my body cooperated or not!
All those things were just moments I had to go through to be the kind of person I am today. So it's all good!

. . . .

Wednesday June 25th, 2008   11:18am

Hello,

I guess I never told you all about my In-laws sending my name in for the Diva of the Day contest. Well, you'll never guess what happened! I won! They made me sound nice and kind of like an angel. I'm thankful that I have cancer and 5 kids. I think that may have moved me to the top of the "Awww" list. There is an article in the June Show Me the Ozarks on me and the contest.

I got to take my friend Margie with me. She is always fun. They put a lot of make up on us. I must say we looked Hot. We also got to ride in this totally cool limo. I felt like we were totally popular, cool girls in high school. We laughed like we were on dentist drugs. Thank you Tonia, Nikki, and Shirley for making me look like I need to be a DIVA for the day!

On another note, there are days when I feel great and other days when I feel 90 years old. I don't want to live to be 90 if this is what it feels like. I mean my knees who have always been there for me before, have without notice gone on vacation. The ones I have now must be some kind of fill-in substitutes. This is not cool! Then of course there is the ever trusting constant stomach ache and everything taste like crap syndrome. Really, I'm not complaining.

I read an article on Dolly Parton one time. (This was a long time ago) She said she stays skinny by just chewing up fattening food and then spitting it out into a cup. After all we only over eat because we like the taste of the food anyway right? When food taste amazing, we eat until we are in pain.

When I first saw that, I thought it was nonsense. I mean I over eat because I have no self-control. Haha. I have realized over these last few months that I am eating just enough to tell my brain that I have actually eaten something. Food either has no taste or a weird taste. My point is, Dolly is right.

Well, I guess I have to pretend I'm cleaning the barn now.

Later taters

. . . .

In the

Home Stretch

I am so proud of all of my kids and how they all helped and dealt with not only the changes I was dealing with but also stepping up and helping when their dad couldn't. The impact this has had on my family has been amazing. We had really started to begin to lean on each other in a way we hadn't before. We had also each begun to lean on God in a way that we hadn't learned to do before. There was a quiet strength in our home.

Most Sundays I couldn't wait to get to church. I needed the worship time. I needed to be in a sanctuary with a hundred other people who were spiritually seeking God and worshiping through music, really feeling his presence.

I am so thankful for God and so thankful for his mercy. I know I am so undeserving.

For God so loved the world that he gave his
one and only Son,
that whoever believes in him shall not perish
but have eternal life

John 3:16

. . . .

Tuesday July 29th, 2008 9:03

Hey all the peeps that I love,

I recently put new photos on the site. I left three old ones though. One to remind me that I look cute with hair too, one to remind me it could be worse and one to remind me that people can love you so much that they go temporarily insane!

I'm sorry I haven't written in a while. Summer gets busy you know? Well, I have had the privilege of seeing many of my family and friends this summer. You just don't realize how much you miss someone, or how dear you hold them in your heart until the moment you want to just get in the car, run to their house and just sit and visit or just hang out for a while. Sometimes we just get busy living though, even if we just live 20 minutes away, that may as well be 20 hours.

I decided to try to do some cleaning the other day. I started in the laundry room. It is decent sized, so I knew it was going to be some work because there are several cabinets full of stuff. I had no idea though, that it would take me almost an entire *day to clean that* one *room. I figured I'd be done by noon at the latest, but that is not at all how it worked out. It seemed like the junk I was sifting through was endless. I kept finding things and saying to myself, "Why is this in here?", "Oh that's where that went to.", and "Good grief, she nearly killed her sister over that and it was right here all along!"*

The summer has of course turned out to be hot and humid. We tried to go enjoy a few days at the lake, and I have to tell you, when the water is warm that can be a little difficult. School is closing in and the thought has made me sad and grateful all at the same time. The kids usually get to a point where they are ready to get back into some form of schedule where their minds and bodies are kept busy.

Well, Thursday is the day. I have to be checked in at KU by 6:30am. They will do a removal of the tumor and any cancer cells and at least one lymph node. I believe God has already taken care of business. As far as I'm concerned, there will be no cancer cells or a need to remove more than the 1st lymph node. I am speaking prophetically, but I believe I Am Cancer Free. I just need to do all this to "sew it all up." So any prayers that you might send up for me, please, please, say them with faith that it is done. And please say thank you on my behalf if you would, that he has been kind and gentle, and merciful.

With all the talk about surgery and such, I have been fielding some fairly blunt questions from my two youngest ones. I have to be careful not to laugh because I know they are obviously very concerned and I don't want to hurt their feelings. It is so hard when your eight year old comes to you with a flush in his cheeks and says, point blank, "Mom are you gonna have one fake boob and one real boob when you come home?" Again, it was hard not to laugh. When I told him that they were just going to take a piece of stuff out of one breast and that I wasn't going to be losing either "boob", he seemed so very relieved. That in itself, made me smile, and thankful for people who love me so much. Just in case you don't spend a lot of time with 8 year old boys, when you say "fake" anything, they are picturing something off the Transformers movie. A boob that transforms! YES! but into what? Maybe it could be an extra hand, cup holder, diaper dispenser, mini mean green machine, fascinating toy, newest electronic device. The possibilities are endless!

I know that you are trying to picture all that, and it's hard.
Well stay cool.
I love ya

. . . .

It's wild how you see things crystal clear when you're not in the middle of a storm any more. It's like having major cloud coverage that blocks all the stars. You don't even realize what is there. Then the clouds clear up. If you live out in the country like we do, when you look up at the sky it is so amazing and so brilliant with all its tiny shining stars, it takes your breath away.

I remember praying and telling myself time after time that there would be nothing but marker. As you will see, my sky was about to clear up.

. . . .

Friday, August 1, 2008   8:48am

Hi,

I got back from K.C. yesterday. I am sore but doing fine. They did say they found some tiny microscopic stuff but not to worry. They got clean margins, and I think I can now say I am CANCER FREE! I had a lot of loved ones who went with me. It was nice to know they were all there. God really is good all the time.

I go back the 7th for a checkup and to see what the next step is. I think we will be getting radiation set up. Thank you again for all your prayers. God heard and blessed me. In return I pray he blesses you!

Love you all
Carol

. . . .

Knowing that the surgery was behind me was a big relief. I was set up to do radiation closer to home. I'm thankful for that. I had to go every day for a couple of months. I'm not sure I was thrilled about that but it is an indication that I was in the home stretch. Friends of mine had assured me that the radiation would be a walk in the park compared to doing the chemo. It was nice to be able to talk to people who have been through it before. It gives you an opportunity to know what to expect.

Summer was coming to a close.

For me it's always a little bit sad to say goodbye to summer. Although I love the fall, its arrival always means that colder weather will be here soon, so I'm always a little bit reluctant to let it go. Fall also means that it's time for the kids to start back to school. Even though it is a little bit of a relief knowing they will be going back, it is again also a little bit sad thinking about the house being empty and quiet again. It is crazy how the house will go from active and crazy to empty and quiet overnight.
With all that being said, it also brings back a sort of normality to life. That is something I think we are all grateful for.

. . . .

Tuesday September 2, 2008 12:39pm

Hey kids,

Well, I'm trying to get this radiation stuff situated so I can get it going. I'm trying to get it all transferred here for obvious reasons. It doesn't make sense to drive two and half hours one way every single day for 2 months when I can drive 20 minutes for the same treatment. Hopefully I can get that worked out this week.

School is back in and the hot weather is starting to let up a bit. Thank you so much for all your support. I have slowly but surely been trying to get out all my thank you cards. I am feeling good and am starting to get some of my hair back! It looks really dark and I guess that's ok but I was hoping it might come back in a little curly. My hair has been straight as a board all my life.

I have so much to tell you but no time to write it. Today is Travis birthday. He is turning 36. I have to go get things to celebrate with!

Talk to you soon

Thursday September 4, 2008 6:57pm

Is it me or do we seriously need a remote control so that we can stop life for a minute so a person can get a handle on things? See I have these teenagers coming, going, and texting me and what not. They are asking questions and when I think I have an answer, they decide they weren't really interested anyway.

But……………… my answer was good!

I made an appointment for my consultation for radiation. I was told it was going to take two hours. What? Two hours? Listen, I have four girls. I can guarantee that we can hash things out and come up with a plan of action inside thirty to forty-five minutes tops. And girls are COMPLICATED. Don't believe me? Just ask me.

Well they are calling me to come watch a movie.

Love you guys

. . . .

The consultation was quite interesting. You lay on a table with your girls hanging out while the doctor puts a laser type grid on you. He then takes this fun little marker and puts tiny little dots in all the right places. After grabbing another doctor to make sure everything looks like I have been sufficiently marked up, we proceed with the next step. The doctor comes at you with what looks like a glorified metal toothpick. He says "little sting." OW! Big sting. Five or so "little stings" later, you are permanently tattooed with these tiny little black pin marks. Why you ask? So they cook only the breast and not your innards. That word makes me laugh. Innards. That's kind of like the word varmint. My mom loves to use that word. For some reason, it always makes me smile.

Alright, back to my point. The consultation was not fun. Interestingly, I now have little tattoos. Does that make me cool?

. . . .

Friday, October 17, 2008   10:23pm

Hey!
It's getting colder. I don't know why. I was perfectly fine with the 70 degree weather.

I was told today I was on my twentieth rads treatment. So after today I think that gives me 13 more treatments. I have to start seeing my radiation dr. every week now I think. This weekly visit has got to be to ensure his new hummer is paid for, because what transpires in these visits are nothing more than him basically saying, "WELL, (in a very thick accent) you tie your shoes so you don't trip yeah?" I nod my head. "WELL. Ok then, see you next week." I'm not kidding. But to be fair I'm not sure if he has a newer hummer. Maybe one of his kids does? That was a joke.

As I told a friend of ours, I shouldn't complain, you know, because I am *alive to do it. The annoying thing about radiation is the every single day thing and the effects it has on your skin. The up side is that they would have freshly baked cookies out every morning. They were so chewy and good!*

I mentioned the effects it has on your skin. (It's cooking it right?) I did something inappropriate in the kitchen this evening. I was scratching the breast. Really, I can't help it. It itches like crazy. When it doesn't itch there is this prickling sensation like someone is poking me with a needle. Travis caught me. He gives me this sideways look and says, "What was that and what are you doing?"

I smile and say I'm sorry, and tell him he is lucky and fortunate. This is because what I really want to do is take the scratchy side of the cheese grater to it. He gives me a look that says "Too much information." Did I already say that it itches?

I'm not sure if I covered this already, but laying there on a steel table with your hands behind your head with your girls out there for everyone to see makes you realize modesty is funny. I lay there thinking, "Boy if the girls at the bingo hall could see me now." They would be jealous I'm sure. This makes me giggle. One of the very sweet ladies that I see everyday up there comes in and joyfully tells me, "Your next!" She then proceeds to tell me that there is a young man in there today that I'll get to look at. The lift of her eyebrows and big smile encourages me. I think "GREAT! And I didn't do my hair! So I get back there to the radiation room and then realize the "young man" she is talking about is older than my dad! Again, this makes me smile. She is so sweet. Monday is her last treatment. She is so excited to be done.

Speaking of Bingo, have you ever been to a bingo hall? Have you ever been friends with a Bingo gamer? If you have not, they are these feisty "older" folks. (Older and younger are relative to our own age aren't they? A lessen I realized in my earlier story) I actually saw a bumper sticker not too long ago that said "Keep an old person off the streets and support your local Bingo hall." I love that. These bingo gamers carry large duffle bag looking things that have approximately 143 dobbers of all colors in them. What's a dobber? It's a giant marker. When you take the cap off the felt tip is flat and the size of a quarter.

If you have never been, I'm going to clue you in. There is very little mercy in VFW bingo. These are pro's. I went with my aunt. I buy two cards thinking I'm big stuff. I have two cards and my very own dobber. I sit down and prepare to kick hinny. All these ladies start sitting down around us with, pause for dramatic effect, five and ten cards! They take all their cards and position them. This is very serious business. They then take five or so dobbers of assorted colors out and line them out in front of them at the top of their cards. I'm sure you can imagine at this point, I am now fearful. I'm deciding this looks like work, not a game.

They start calling. This is NOT the PTA bingo I know. They are calling them fast! These older ladies who can't drive faster than 35 in a 45 are checking and marking ten cards in less time than I can mark my two cards! I also learned in this trip that you can get Bingo with all sorts of things other than straight or diagonal. There's "corners," the "X "and then the ultimate, the "black out." So to shorten my long story, I win. The problem though is that I did not take note of the ladies around me when they were pulling all their cards apart. I yell Bingo. They are all looking at me like, YEAH? My aunt then says, "Tear it off and hold it up!" Finally hastily, I get that done and hold it up. The announcer then says

"You have to hold it up and say Bingo at the same time." Really? Well, good grief. I think the lady across from me and the lady two tables over were thinking, "Young kid comes in here, she can't hardly keep up and doesn't know the rules, she is lucky I have a bad hip!" I guess I don't really have to tell you what I did next. I grabbed the money and ran.

The moral of the story is Bingo can be very exciting. Older ladies are very competitive. Don't sit by someone who has a cane. Especially a very nice ornate cane, those can leave a mark!

I want to share with you all some pretty cool things God has been doing in our lives but it is getting late, so I will have to save it for next time. In the meantime don't forget October is breast cancer awareness month. Wear Pink! Do a self-exam and get anything checked out that seems off or strange and pray for everyone who lifes it may have already touched.

May God touch <u>you</u> *and make* <u>you</u> *a light in the world!*

Love ya,
Carol

P.S. Did you know that very few doctors specialize in this field because of the difficulties in diagnosis and resulting law suits? 55 percent of all breast cancer specialists have had a suit brought against them. It's just something to think about.

. . . .

Radiation is a bit like going in and getting microwaved, or being "nuked" as we call it at our house.

The whole radiation thing was every stinkin day. Sometimes it seemed like a whole lot of trouble for nothing. I would drive about twenty five minutes to the doctor's office then take about 10 minutes getting undressed, five minutes getting nuked, then dressed and back home again. This was every day for at least a month and a half.

It's funny, because if you think of radiation in every day terms it really brings home what it is doing. For instance I know if I am trying to thaw out some meat in the microwave, it thaws pretty quickly. We all know that if it goes too long in the microwave, it not only thaws it, it cooks it. You ever cooked meat in the microwave a little too long? Yeah, it's not good. So the whole time I'm laying on that table being "nuked", I'm just thinking "Lord, please let them be aiming at the right place and please make sure the timer is set right."

I'm not sure what a solid cooked breast would look like next to the other but, I am pretty sure needing a bra for that side would no longer be an issue.

I'm sure you have picked up by now that I did not lose my breast. This is because my doctor chose according to my kind of cancer and tumor size, to do chemo first. The chemo shrunk the tumor to microscopic size. By the naked eye, by time they went in to do the surgery, all they could see was the marker they placed in the middle of the tumor. They did what they call breast conserving surgery. They took margins around the tumor to make sure they got all the cancer, and that's it. Can you tell? Yeah, a little, but you would really have to look. The two, two inch scars kind of give it away, but that's something I can definitely live with. I have another scar kind of closer to my collar bone where my port was at. I tease my husband and tell him I'm gonna go get a tattoo of lips over it with the words "Cancer Goodbye". You know, as in kiss cancer goodbye. I thought it was funny. My husband just raised one eyebrow and said "If that's what you think you need to do." Maybe I should have suggested matching tattoos.

You know how we were talking about radiation and how it's kind of like being nuked or microwaved? Well, I started to see the effects of the treatments about halfway through. My skin started itching like crazy. It got red and irritated. At first it sort of felt like a really bad sun burn. I guess that's what it's like to be cooked very slowly.
I was told to put thick layers of lotion on. It didn't really help. I am really very fair skinned though. Maybe because I'm almost translucent it cooked faster. (That's supposed to be funny.)

I'm on the other side of it now. I am so very thankful we didn't really have any glitches. I'm pretty much healed and starting to feel somewhat normal again.

. . . .

Monday February 2, 2009   8:55am

Good morning! I thought I would update all the people I love. It has been six months and I am still cancer free! It all seems like a distant memory. It was just here, and then it was gone. It's strange how life works like that.

I have been a little freaked out about the things we put in our body and how we get cancer and all that, so I decided on a New Year's resolution. I have decided not to eat meat for a month. It's funny, because for some reason this was very hard on my family. Now, just so you know, I did not ask them to go meatless as this was my resolution not theirs. I didn't think it was fair to torture them too.

They were cracking me up. I have never seen such craziness. You would think I was some high official they were trying to schmooze to get me to vote their way. I'm not sure but I was beginning to think they were all getting kickbacks from the "American Meat Council" for all their constant plugs. They were pushing meat like some kind of back alley drug pusher. I think you all would have been proud of me. Like the sign says, I just kept saying No!

How did it go you ask? Well, it's not been too bad. I learned there are a lot of things you can eat that does not include meat. Unfortunately some of the best comfort foods include meat, so that part was a little rough. (I just need to say here, I love and missed Wendy's chili, and that doesn't even touch roasts, homemade chicken and noodles, and some of my mother-in-laws meatloaf) We went to dinner at friends' houses, and you know they went out of their way to have something that I could eat as well. They were very thoughtful and sweet. (Thank you Carolyn and Carrie.) So I guess to sum it up, I learned a lot about many things surrounding this month long journey. I'm glad I did it. I know for sure now, I am a carnivore through and through.

Well I hope to give you updates in another six months to let you know that I am still cancer free.
I hope this finds you all well.

Love
Carol

. . . .

I continue to look back and see where God was. I can look back and see him in the moments I was worried. I am amazed at how he moves when we let go of ourselves and allow him to take what we can't carry. I wonder what happens when you don't know how to do that?

He reached down from on high and

Took hold of me;

He drew me out of deep waters

.

He rescued me from my powerful enemy;

From my foes, who were too strong for me.

They confronted me in the day

Of my disaster,

But the Lord was my support.

He brought me out into

A spacious place;

He rescued me because he delighted in me.

Psalms 18:16-19

The emphasis on verse 17 is mine. “He rescued me from my powerful enemy; from my foes, *who were too strong for me.* How many times have we felt like we were fighting a current, an unseen thing, that felt too strong for us? I know I have many times. Cancer was another unseen thing. We think we can handle them on our own and we try to, don’t we? We try to be big boys and girls and do what we think is Sometimes though, whatever we are going through isn't going to be a quick fix. Sometimes it isn't even something we can do on our own. It is only when we give up ourselves and lay everything at Gods feet, in faith, that something changes. I knew from the beginning, cancer was not something I could do in any way shape or form without God. So I laid it at his feet and did what the doctors said. I walked in total faith that he had total control. It released me from so much. All I had to do was pray and follow directions.

Nothing to it.

. . . .

Tuesday April 21, 2009   11:11pm

Hello all,

I wanted to give you all one last update before I deleted this account.

I am still cancer free! Nine months this month. I will go for another checkup in August which will make it a year. A YEAR! Do you know how amazing that is? It makes me think of that song, how's it go? "God of mercy humbled I bow down,……I called… you answered, you came to my rescue, and I want be where you are." I have looked back over the last year many times and think how amazing it all is. All of that brings another song to mind, "In my life be lifted high, in my world be lifted high, in my love be lifted high."

Thank you to everyone who read my craziness. Thank you all for reading through my typo's, for signing my guestbook with so many encouraging words, for loving on me and my family, for praying for us, sending monetary gifts, and for continually keeping us close in heart.

I have enjoyed writing and reading your feedback. I hope to write or blog again on something entirely different.

For the record for those of you who have not seen me in a while, I do actually have some hair. It is hard to be in this in-between stage, but then I go back and look at pictures and think, "No, that *was a little more irritating."*
So I guess as they say, it's all in levels.

I love you all, and thank you so much for being there for me.

Love Carol

The Support

I wanted to show you the support I had while I was going through all this. These are a few of my guestbook entries. I love them all and am so thankful for each person who took the time to write. They helped me get through some pretty long nights.

Colossians 3:12-14

Put on then, as God's chosen ones, holy and beloved, compassionate hearts, kindness, humility, meekness, and patience, bearing with one another and, if one has a complaint against another, forgiving each other; as the Lord has forgiven you, so you also must forgive. And above all these put on love, which binds everything together in perfect harmony.

March 18th 2008

Carol,

Glad you are home tonight. It is good to come home and be with your family. We are so proud of you. Your faith in our Lord is the first thing you have, and then there is your family, extended family, and then friends. We love you and you little family is in our prayers. "Where more than one gathers in my name" and we love you!! Mom

Shirley Mondt

March 20th 2008

Carol,

I am Travis's second cousin. I don't think I have had the opportunity to meet you. When Shirley started putting out the word for prayer, I put you on my daily prayer list. I lift you up daily to our precious God. He is holding you in HIS arms and He will bring you through this struggle.

We can call on Jesus any time of the night or day.
He's always there waiting for our call. What a blessing that is!
No phone needed, no e-mails, just a whisper.

Don't be afraid to be human, God understands you completely and you are always in his presence.

"My grace is sufficient for you, for My strength is made perfect in weakness"

2 Corinthians 12:9-10

Tosh

March 28, 2008

Carol,

Just read your latest journal entry and you had me laughing. Imagine it…… Feeling tired after spending the day caring for your mom's needs, then reading some of your experiences of the day had me joining in visualizing your predicament and finding humor and a smile too. You are something and I believe you have definitely found a way to fight this cancer head on with as much humor as you can muster. Laughter is healing and if it helps you to look for the funny stuff, this may be the greatest stress reliever! You must have had this quality before cancer ever entered your lifestyle. That is one big plus for you and your family. Just thinking about you and sending hugs from Texas.

Janis Watson

March 29, 2008

Carol,

I haven't been through the treatments you have been going through, but I am a seven year breast cancer survivor and I know if you trust in God, keep the right attitude, and do your best God will take care of you. He is an awesome God. Keep your sense of humor.

Shirley Randleman

March 31, 2008

You are wonderful! We really appreciate your humor! Thanks for having cancer and making us laugh!! ☺

Rick Harter

April 1, 2008

Good morning Aunt Carol. How did you sleep? I love and miss you!

Love you

Taya

April 1, 2008

Carol,

Hey girl! I just want to let you know that I love you! I am sorry you are going through this. We are all praying for ya and rooting for ya, so hang in there. If you need someone to talk to, you can always call or email me. You do have a great attitude about this and life. I think that is awesome! So rock on chicky!
Love your oldest but youngest looking cousin.

Daniele

April 1, 2008

Carol,

I always look forward to your journal entries. You have a tremendous sense of humor. I'm sure you have your down times but you sure know how to look at the bright side of things.

Most people don't have your good attitude when they don't have any real problems in life. You make all of us smile when we read what you write. We should be cheering you up, instead you are cheering us up. You're amazing and I think you are pretty special person. I know God has you in his hands.

Tosh

April 2, 2008

Carol,

You have been on my mind a lot and I love your positive attitude and humor. You have your faith in God, a positive attitude, your humor, your family on both sides and friends that love and pray for you. I know you are hearing from many earth angels as I call them, that are there for you and yours either by this, phone, cards, the ones that help in one form or another such as meals or the nurses or Drs at the hospital and it is overwhelming how many you have and all that God has provided for you to get you through this.

Blessings to you,

Love Trudy

April 3, 2008

As I glance from time to time at our journal, I am reminded that God is indeed in the blessing business! I don't pretend to know why you are going through this at this time, or even why it had to be you but I rest assured in the knowledge that God knows! You are a great source of inspiration to all who have come to know you whether it be through your blog, or through family. I am uplifted and encouraged to know you, and not really know you (not having met you), but you give my spirit great joy and hope!!

They say everything happens for a reason, (and I am sure you are tired of hearing that), but I sure feel blessed by you.

God is working through you to touch other people and give them hope in their time of need. (I know you say choose someone else right?) So I say Thank You to GOD and to you for renewing my hope, trust, and faith that no matter what we are going through in this life, GOD has not forgotten us and this battle is not ours, it's the Lord's! THANK YOU!

Melodee Colbert

April 3, 2008

Hey Carol,

Just wanted to say we love you. You are an absolute inspiration. Thank you.

Love you,

Lisa Comer

April 4, 2008

Carol,

You are amazing. I can't believe the spirit you have in knowing what you are going to go through. Well, it's the Lord by your side huh? I have a little story to tell you about a friend I worked with about 28 years ago.

There was a lady named Bonnie who was in my dept. She got breast cancer. During her chemo she would come back to work and she would ask me if she could lay her head down on her work table. She had to work. I said yes of course. She had it really bad. A few months ago I was in line at the store and someone said, "Donna is that you?" I turned around and there was Bonnie and her granddaughter. She looked wonderful. I retired before I knew what happened to her. See how God works, so you can trust in him and you will be fine. You are in my prayers every day.

Love, Donna

April 4, 2008

Well today I got in your guestbook!

I really miss the time we used to spend together.
You have always had such great strength in anything you have wanted to do. Even those things that you detest doing you carry through it and get it done with pride.

God has given you such a gift of caring, loving, patience, and laughter. You can see your personality as I call them (gifts) carried over into your great bunch of children and the peace your husband has on his face when he talks about his wife. You can tell in his voice you mean everything to him. How you are blessed!!!

Love to you all

Leslie Chasten

April 8, 2008

Just wanted you to know that you and your family are in our prayers. You are a wonderful person and I know you will beat this. If you need anything give us a hollar.

Love you all…………………kisses

Becky Woody

April 10, 2008

I sure love you guys! You guys are meant for each other. Keeping light of everything is great. Not only do we need light and guidance from our Father, (God) which we are so blessed to get, but you also have the light and guidance from each other. With a wonderful family standing beside you, including your children!

I thank the father every day for the light he gives us and the blessings he gives us. One of the things I thank him most for is our health. I thank him for your health and the healing that is taking place in your body. Like Travis said we are his children and he cares for us very much, more than anyone else.

I have no doubt in faith, or our father that my cousin is a wonderful mother, cousin, woman and person, that you're healed. Confessing is the first step to believing.

Love you all very much. Can't wait to see you!

Love Tonia

April 12, 2008

Hi Carol,

Just wanted to write a few words to tell you how much you inspire me. You are a terrific testimony of the strength God gives his people. I know he smiles as he watches you face each new day with the courage he provides for you.

I am doing a Beth Moore series called "Jesus the One and Only". It is fabulous and has given me fresh insight to who he is and what he wants for his children. Something she said that made such an impression on me and made me think of you almost instantly. She liked God's protection to an umbrella. When storms come our way and we trust him, we remain under his umbrella…… we can STILL dance in the rain. Is that just like our God or what?!?!?!

That is you my sweet sister….you are dancing in the rain, under the umbrella that he has provided just for you. Even when the storms seem almost too much to stand against…you dance. I so admire your strength and awesome faith. I know he is watching over you and holding that umbrella high.

I love you! Keep dancing!

Rochelle Doss

April 13, 2008

Carol,

The hat party was great! Your laughter and high spirits were a blessing to all who attended. Ya'll have so many friends and family who love you so very much. It was good to see you feeling so much better. It is so amazing to watch you spring back to your old bubbly self after each treatment. I can't help myself from worrying about you but you always seem to show me that I worry too much.

I believe you and Travis are truly angels on earth. My opinion is not just a mothers prejudice, God knows you are his angels and will take all the dark clouds away when the time is right. All of this is temporary. I believe it is Gods way of bringing all your family (uncles aunts cousins) back together stronger than before.
You. Travis Nychelle, Brice, Alexandria, Alaina, and Noah are such strong witnesses for God's glory that he seeing you through this trial to witness your faith to everyone around you in a way only angels can.

So in closing keep you faith strong, you head high, and your smile bright. Always know that you are loved and that god is holding you and your family in his arms as a parent does with their new born baby.

Love you always,

Mom

April 17, 2008

We've never met before. I am Travis' second cousin.
Your lovely attitude toward ending this awful disease is so endearing. I know you must have times that you find it hard to have humor in, but just keep looking up. And if you get discouraged about the effects of the meds on your face, just remember that God only looks at our hearts.

I can tell by reading that all of these people love you so much and that they only see your heart too. It shows in your attitude and humor.

No wonder you have a huge support group. I will pray for your strength through this trial, that you will find comfort and that you will continue to find joy.

In Christ, Jo Josephson

April 18, 2008

Carol,

This is your husband! I was reading and realize there wasn't anything from me on here, so I thought I would write something to you. I will make this short and sweet. Anything I can say would be ultimately summed up in these words alone…

I LOVE YOU!
The lord sees your faith and will heal you.

There is absolutely nothing too big for our Lord. He will resolve all these issues. We will revisit them from time to time in the future as we move onward through this foggy world, using these experiences to help others.

Once again, I want you to know,
I LOVE YOU!!!

One other thing, I know I told you before, But I will tell you and everyone again now…….

Do NOT be discouraged by how you appear right now or anytime because I always see you as Carol, my wife. It wouldn't matter to me if you were completely unrecognizable. If I know it is you, I cannot love you anymore than I do right now.

I see you as 200% B-E-A-U-T-I-F-U-L.
When I see you, I truly see you as I always have. Knowing you are near me makes me calm and more myself than anything in this world.
OK, so it wasn't short!

Travis Goad

April 25, 2008

Carol and Travis,

Just wanted to say I just spoke with Binda about your benefit. You have a wonderful friend in that lady! Just speaking to her I could tell that she truly loves you as all of us do. Hope to see your smiling face soon. Want to let you know that you are in our prayers. I just know there is going to be GOOOD news soon!

With all our love,

Brenda and Wayne.

May 5, 2008

It's been awhile since I have written to you....After reading what you posted, I am in tears. No really I am...I just took lunch and checked my email. I am so sorry that I couldn't be there Saturday.
I see God working in such a mighty way. I am proud of you and the stance you have taken....I have peace knowing your love of Christ and that you do not blame him for this affliction. That you are standing tall knowing that he has gone before you, making the way, every step. I love and adore you.
I find strength in what you write and feel as though I fail you. I should be lifting you up, yet it's the other way around. My apologies for this. Carol....you're an angel of the Lord. Times will be trying, Satan will attack...we have the power to defend our family and to go to battle for one another, in the name of Jesus. The people he has placed in your life to help you walk this journey, I pray for blessings on them. They are fighting with you, crying out to God on your behalf. I would like to say "THANK YOU" to all of you who join her in this season of life. Your prayers hold more power then you know. When two or three come together in my name....I cling to this often.

Not that I need to...but to touch on what you said about missing your Dad. This is something that many of us suffer from. He is PROUD, he does LOVE you, and he is waiting for you to rejoice, so that on a bright sunny day, when we are all just sitting around.....doing nothing. talking about everything and nothing at all...(man we are so good at that nothing part)...he will be there Carol. I promise...in the midst of it all. We shall see him again someday. I know this is true

Love you

Jamie Everett

MAY 15, 2008

Good morning honey:

I am so glad you have been feeling at least decent for the past several days, and I know you are dreading your trip to KU med Monday for treatments. Your courage and lightheartedness has astounded and warmed the hearts of so many. You looked so pretty Tuesday, and of course Travis was so handsome, and I never even got a picture.

You are like an Eagle soaring high in the heavens and gliding along. Your strength and faith in our precious Savior I know, has carried you through all of this and He will continue to do so. I am so blessed to have you in the family. You have done and done for me and now it is my turn.

Love to you on this day that God has set aside for all to absorb and be glad in. Mom

Shirley Mondt

JUNE 25, 2008

LOL!! I was just thinking a few minutes ago that I hadn't seen anything posted in a while. You always make me laugh. I hope your knees come back home soon. Hopefully, they don't "look" 90 years old, too. :)
I love you. Call me sometime!
BTW, where is my birthday card? You know it's been a month now, right...
Love you,

Misti Millsap

August 1, 2008

Hello Carol,

This is Robert Doss and Deborah,

We are truly happy for you. We hope and pray all things just keep getting better each and every day for you and yours. Tell Travis I said hi and God Bless

Robert Doss

*****As I was proof reading and going over these notes from everyone, I became emotional. During the time that I was going through treatment I was trying to concentrate on pushing through. But now I realize the true impact of their words. Obviously I had read them before, but this time it was as if their love, hope and support leaped off the page.

All I can think is, WOW! How blessed am I?

Epilogue

I hope you enjoyed this book. My intention was to tell my story and in the process give encouragement. My hope is that you will pass this book on to someone else who could use the information and encouragement as well.

Many times while I was in the process of writing this book I came upon someone who was scheduled for a biopsy, or someone who was already doing treatment. I was so frustrated because there was so much I wanted to share. At the time I just kept saying to myself, I wish I had this book done so I could just hand it to them. I told my husband that if nothing ever comes of this but the opportunity to hand it out to women who are scared and in need of a laugh, it will have served its purpose.

I love that God has blessed me with this opportunity as well as the blessings you will receive if you get a chance to pass this book on. God works in mighty ways when we allow him to walk through our pain and troubles with us. He helps us grow through his grace and mercy. How awesome is that?

I would love to hear your feedback.
Please send me an e-mail to;
c_goad@live.com

Thank You for reading, buying and passing along this book. *The fact that you are holding this book in your hands is not an accident.* I can't help but believe God is in the middle of it, and in the middle of you.

Till next time,

Matthew 22:36-40

With love,
Carol Goad

*You can order more copies of this book at -

www.BuyBooksontheWeb.com

Made in the USA
Monee, IL
04 November 2026

67381744R10079